The future *Breakthrough* takes us on a fascinating tour of the medical, scientific, and technological advances predicted in our lifetime that will alter the way we live.

These breakthroughs are miraculous! From improving our health and increasing longevity to providing a keener understanding of the universe, the book is studded with exciting discoveries—tests, cures, devices, processes, and theories—certain to enrich our lives.

Charles Panati is an ideal guide. He has been head physicist at RCA and a science editor at *Newsweek*. His excitement is contagious. His presentation is characterized by energy, clarity, and resolute optimism for the decades ahead. In this era of faulting medicine, science, and technology for shortcomings, he reminds us of the infinite ways they enhance contemporary life.

Whether reading the book straight through or browsing among various chapters and thirty-three witty illustrations, the reader is guaranteed an entrancing and hopeful exploration of the future. *Breakthroughs* is the perfect way to prepare yourself for the wondrous events of the 1980s and 1990s.

BREAKTHROUGHS

Books by Charles Panati

Supersenses
The Geller Papers (editor)
Links
Breakthroughs

BREAKTHROUGHS

Astonishing Advances in Your
Lifetime in Medicine, Science,
and Technology

Charles Panati

Illustrations by Stan Fedinick

Houghton Mifflin Company Boston 1980

Library of Congress Cataloging in Publication Data

Panati, Charles, date
    Breakthroughs.

    Includes bibliographical references.
    1. Medicine—History—20th century.
2. Medical innovations. 3. Technological
innovations. I. Title.
R149.P36   610'.9'04   79-26269
ISBN 0-395-28221-7

Printed in the United States of America
v 10 9 8 7 6 5 4 3 2 1

The author is grateful for permission to use the
chart in the chapter "Aging Breakthroughs." It is
reprinted from *The Futurist* (June 1978), published
by the World Future Society.

Portions of this book have appeared in *Science Digest*.

For my aunts
  FAY, KAY, ANNE, AND THELMA
and uncles
  CARL, ANGE, AND BOB

Special thanks to Michael Hudson for his helpful suggestions
and editing, to Stan Fedinick for the style and imagination
he brought to the drawings, and to my mother for her consci-
entious typing of the manuscript.

Contents

PART III · TECHNOLOGY

Part I

Medicine

1

Holistic Health Breakthroughs:
Your Mind as Healer–and Slayer

Treating the Whole You

Your state of mind can make you sick or speed your recovery from illness. The idea is hardly new, but only now is it gaining the attention and respect of Western doctors. The result is a variety of new medical therapies that are being developed for the 1980s and 1990s. This approach, called holistic medicine, is based on four general principles:

• Your mind and body are inseparable. Therefore, not just the disease itself must be treated, but the entire you. This may entail having to change your self-image and your outlook on the future, as well as on your immediate disease.

• You have the power to heal yourself and the power to remain well. This "power" also involves the *will power* to treat your body to wholesome eating, drinking, and living.

• A positive, supportive relationship between you and your doctor can be more beneficial than drugs in curing diseases, particularly mental ones.

• Emphasis should be placed on preventive medicine through a better understanding of nutrition and a healthful life style.

Dr. Jerome Frank, professor emeritus of psychiatry at the Johns Hopkins School of Medicine, has studied the mind-health connection and documented many cases that illustrate how the mind can play the major — or sole — role in a cure.

Drugs

Several studies reveal that drugs will often perform according to a person's expectations. Psychiatric patients at one major hospital were divided into two groups. One group received the tranquilizer Stelazine while members of the other group were given a placebo. The experiment was "double blind" in that neither the doctors nor the patients knew who received the drug. Surprisingly, slightly *more* patients were tranquilized by the placebo than by Stelazine. The experiment was then repeated and the patients were given double doses and told that the additional dosage would accelerate their reaction to the medication. With uncanny precision, almost twice the number in each group became docile in half the time. Those taking a double dose of the placebo acted more relaxed than those receiving a double dose of the actual drug. Commenting on the results, Dr. Frank wrote, in *Human Nature*, "The studies indicate that in many cases, particularly in those involving a person's state of mind, the effect of medication is influenced by the hope of cure, coupled with a belief in the physician, who in some unknown way conveys his sense of the strength and effectiveness of the drug."

Disease

In another hospital three women patients who had not responded to conventional treatment for pancreatitis, gall-bladder surgery, and cancer were visited by a faith healer disguised as a doctor. He performed his psychic ministrations without informing the women of his true identity, and after twelve sessions none of the patients showed improvement. They were then informed that a famous faith healer would be working on them from his home every morning for three days — when in fact he was not going to do so. The results this time were astonishing. One skinny, bedridden woman got up and walked after the first "session" — and in a few weeks gained thirty pounds. After the second "treatment" the cancer patient's red blood cell count rose and she was strong enough to return home, where she died months later. In fact all three women felt better and left the hospital in a week's time. They had experienced real physical improvements, which had been self-induced.

Miracles

We often describe a shattered love affair as resulting in a broken heart, and there may be more truth to those words than we ever conjectured. Studies reveal that of all our body organs the heart may be the most susceptible to emotional influence. In one test involving a heart patient suffering from angina, a leading surgeon performed a fake operation by opening the patient's chest but not taking any surgical steps to remedy the ailment. Yet after recovering from what he thought was major surgery, the patient reported a reduction in anginal pain, and he was able to resume an active, full life. The surgeon concluded that the mock operation proved every bit as effective as actual heart surgery. We may cure ourselves more often than we think. "State of mind may well account for the 'miracle' cures reported at healing shrines such as Lourdes," Dr. Frank observes. "The cures are not really miraculous in that they defy natural laws. They are followed by normal, though rapid, healing processes. Tissue healing, for instance, takes place over a period of days or weeks." (See *Biofeedback for Your Heart*, p. 48.)

Environment

The surroundings in which you recover from an illness can also be important. A team of doctors and health experts recently transformed a Veterans' Administration hospital from a bleak building that once housed patients in crowded, colorless cubicles into a bright, cheerful hospital. Doctors expected some improvement in their patients but were astonished by the high incidence of recuperation. Within three months many patients who had been hospitalized from three to ten years not only were healthy enough to be discharged, but once discharged resumed normal lives. "We have seen the importance of treating the sick person as a totality," says Dr. Frank, "not just as a body in need of repair. This unified system of healing should be our ultimate goal."

•   •   •

So vital is the mind-body interaction that the World Health Organization has recommended that in certain instances Western doctors practicing in Third World countries might have greater success if on their rounds they were accompanied by the country's traditional healers — shamans, sorcerers, witch doctors, and midwives.

Where a physician once healed the body, a psychiatrist the head, and a clergyman the soul, the holistic doctors of the 1980s and 1990s will be required to play all three roles. And for the first time in the history of medicine you as the patient will be expected to participate actively in the healing process. In the section that follows we will examine new mind-body therapies that may become a reality in your lifetime.

Touch Me, Heal Me

We realize that the human touch soothes, but it may also heal. In the future, doctors and nurses may be trained to hold their patients' hands or stroke their patients' injuries. In this way parents and children and spouses may to some extent become general physicians at home.

At the University of Maryland Medical School, Dr. James Lynch, a specialist in psychosomatic medicine, has found that petting animals has a beneficial effect on their cardiovascular system; it also increases their resistance to infections. Similar results are being observed with human patients: even people in deep comas often register improved heart rate and brainwaves when their hands are held by doctors, nurses, or family members. Dr. Lynch extrapolates these early findings for a broad human base. "There is a biological basis for our need to form human relationships," he says. "If we fail to fulfill that need, our health is in peril."

Although those biological foundations have yet to be discovered, one new medical treatment called therapeutic touch is gradually being introduced into hospitals and nursing schools around the country. Simply stated, nurses attempt to make sick patients feel better by a sort of "laying on of hands." Pioneered by Dr. Dolores Krieger of New York University's School of Nursing, the therapy creates a physical closeness between two people, even though the nurse never touches the patient but holds her hands about an inch above the patient's body (and not always the ailing part). Dr. Krieger suspects that the treating nurse actually transmits energy to the patient, which aids in recovery. Medical authorities are skeptical of that claim but agree that in many cases therapeutic touch works. Stroking a fevered forehead, holding the hand of a suffering patient, or merely sitting by a patient's bed — such a therapeutic touch may work simply because it raises the patient's spirits and, as a result, the bodily defenses. As holistic medicine teaches, anything that makes you feel better can also influence your recovery.

So far more than 3000 doctors, nurses, therapists, and even some veterinarians have mastered the technique of therapeutic touch, and their number is steadily growing. More hospitals are permitting their staffs to practice the treatment as an adjunct to — never in place of — conventional therapies. Only future experiments will determine whether touching heals for physical or psychological reasons. In the meantime, we may see physicians in the 1980s and 1990s prescribing less medication and dispensing a lot more Tender Loving Care.

A Measure of Faith

Why do sugar pills, or placebos, produce almost immediate relief from pain for many people who take them? Of course, the people using the pills believe they are actual painkillers. But there's much more to the placebo effect than that. The discovery of a new link between the belief that a sugar pill will work and subsequent changes in brain chemistry promises to open new areas in the treatment of pain.

Modern doctors have repeatedly verified a fact familiar to every witch doctor: if a patient is convinced that a treatment will work, it often does. Medical experiments are probing the mysterious mechanism underlying this effect. It is not just the patient's mental attitude that's affected: placebos not only relieve pain but have cured such ills as stomach ulcers, burns, and infections. Further, if you take a large enough sampling of people suffering a common complaint and administer placebos, you can reliably predict that almost exactly a third of them will react positively to the bogus pills. What is the effect of placebos on the body? And why is it that a constant third of the population is always fooled?

Doctors have begun to answer at least the first question. In 1977 researchers at the University of California discovered that several patients given placebos were able subconsciously to activate their body's own pain-suppression system: their brains released more of the natural opiates called enkephalins and endorphins, which, among other functions, act like morphine. Patients who reported the greatest relief from pain were found to have produced the highest amounts of brain opiates. In fact, the amount of these chemicals released may be a measure of just how much faith you have in your doctor and his medication.

The California scientists are the first to document a biochemical basis for the placebo effect. They hope eventually to determine the pathway — from neuron to neuron — by which faith activates chemical production in the brain. It may be that a person convinced of the beneficial effects of a pill (or medical treatment) transmits the message to the brain cells that affect the injured part of the body, and the brain cells in turn behave in such a way as to duplicate the effect of real medication. Pinpointing faith to a biological procedure would go a long way in explaining how the mind influences our health.

And why do almost exactly one third of the patients respond favorably to the sugar pills? Perhaps in discovering the pathway from belief to brain chemistry doctors will learn why a "gullible" one third of the population is always fooled by sugar pills, but a "skeptical" two-thirds continue to suffer.

The Mind-Cancer Link

If you occasionally shout at your children, tell off the boss, and treat yourself to a hearty cry, those around you may tire of these emotional outbursts but you may be healthier for not suppressing your feelings. You may, in fact, substantially lower your risk of developing cancer.

As the mind can help heal the body, it can also contribute to its decline into serious illness. The second-century physician Galen claimed that women with melancholic personalities were more susceptible to breast cancer than those of a sanguine bent, and he may have been right. Doctors are learning that people (particularly women) who for years nurse the grudge that they are victimized by life, repress anger, deny true emotions, or can't cope with traumatic experiences run a greater risk of developing cancer. The evidence for a mind-cancer link remains sparse but is growing steadily stronger. Thus far doctors have established these connections:

• At the National Cancer Institute scientists have found that patients with certain personality traits run a higher risk of suffering a second bout with cancer. Among a large group of patients successfully operated on for malignant tumors, those who relapsed most frequently were repressed, saturnine individuals, who denied feelings of anger and scoffed at the seriousness of their illnesses.

• A decade ago NCI scientists proved the link between smoking and lung cancer; today they are learning that certain smokers run a higher risk than others. Researchers found that the more emotionally repressed a smoker was, the fewer the cigarettes required to induce lung cancer in that person.

• The mind-cancer link may be more tightly forged in women than in men. At the University of Rochester, Dr. Arthur Schmale administered psychological tests to fifty-one women suspected of having cervical cancer. Scoring the tests based on feelings of hopelessness and recent emotional loss, Schmale correctly identified thirty-six women who on further examination were found to have cancer. Doctors at Kings College Hospital in London have observed that a factor common to women they were treating for breast cancer was the inability to vent anger. This finding has just recently been confirmed — and amplified — by doctors at the Johns Hopkins School of Medicine: women with breast cancer who express a high degree of anger toward their disease, their doctors, and their families live longer than those who are pliant, cooperative, or deny concern for their illness.

Imagery Therapy

The connection between cancer and repressed emotions, especially anger, is graphically illustrated by the work of Texas researcher Dr. Carl Simonton. Simonton asks his patients to visualize and draw pictures of their cancer, then encourages them to imagine their white blood cells attacking and eating the cancer cells. Simonton's basic idea is to help people gain a sense of control over what's happening to their bodies. The imagery is thought to be a very sensitive reflection of a patient's emotional state and, therefore, of his or her prospects for improvement. Interestingly, people who can't envisage their white cells as aggressors also have difficulty expressing anger in real-life situations. And their response to visualization combined with conventional cancer therapy is poor.

Perhaps one of the most amazing cases that illustrates the power of the mind over body was reported by Dr. Bruno Klopfer. A man with advanced lymphatic cancer was included in an experimental study of the since-discredited drug Krebiozen. After one dose, his tumors disappeared and he regained enough strength to walk. When the first published reports claimed that the drug was ineffective, the tumors returned and he became bedridden. His physician, in a last-ditch effort to save him, told him the reports were false and treated him with "double strength" Krebiozen — actually, an injection of water. The man again experienced rapid remission. Finally, the American Medical Association and the Food and Drug Administration pronounced the drug worthless, and the man died a few days later.

Doctors believe that it will be at least a decade before they understand the biochemistry of the mind-cancer link. Hormones, antibodies, and even the brain's neurotransmitters are suspected to play a role. (See Chapter 3, Cancer Breakthroughs.) Meanwhile, NCI scientists hope to produce a list of behavioral traits and personality types who have a propensity toward cancer: a sort of "cancer profile." It may be possible to identify these individuals in adolescence or even in childhood. A child who always represses emotions and has a negative self-image could be helped through behavioral therapy or psychotherapy, and possibly avoid developing cancer later in life.

The Mind-Heart Link

A young, healthy person who exercises every day may nevertheless die suddenly from a heart attack. The autopsy may reveal no blocked arteries. In fact, all evidence may indicate that the heart pumped robustly right up to the moment of the attack. This type of heart attack is on the rise.

Doctors have assumed that such mysterious deaths were due to a subtle ailment they had not yet either discovered in the individual or identified in the general population. But according to studies, the anatomical culprit of death is not the heart; it is the brain. Dr. James Skinner of the Baylor University College of Medicine asserts that the fatal link between the two organs is how a person copes with stress. Doctors know that the brain regulates changes in respiration and heart rate. When an animal fights or flees from a life-threatening situation, it's the brain that orders the heart to pump faster. In modern man, Skinner believes, this "cerebral defense system" is activated by stress, and the three most dangerous "stressors" (stress-causing events) are marital strife, job insecurity, and bereavement. The brain recognizes stress, monitors it over weeks or years, and when some level of critical tolerance is reached, it shocks the heart into fatal fibrillations.

Scientists are just beginning to map the stress route from the brain to the heart. At the University of California at Los Angeles, researchers have demonstrated that electrical stimulation to one part of the brain causes irreversible damage to the heart, even though it elicits no behavioral response. At the University of Virginia School of Medicine, Dr. David Cohen is learning that stimulation of other nerve cells in the brain causes a drop in blood pressure to a fatal low. There is preliminary evidence that an increase in the brain chemical serotonin (which acts, among its many roles, as a natural tranquilizer and sleeping pill) decreases the heart's vulnerability to stress. Dr. Cohen believes that serotonin may be the clue to the production of a drug that would reduce the impact of stress. Skinner, on the other hand, believes the development of the ultimate antistress pill may come from studies of other brain chemicals that are just now being identified as having an effect on the heart. "First we must understand the functioning before we know which drug to use," he says. "Then we could develop a pill that would enable people to lessen their cardiac vulnerability without moving back into the jungle."

Since such a pill is at least a decade away, our best course currently is to avoid stressful situations whenever possible, especially marital strife, which seems to be particularly dangerous. Remember, the heart rules the head in matters of love, but when it comes to grief, it's the head that rules the heart.

2

Nutrition Breakthroughs:
What–and How–You'll Eat. And Why

Your Own Computer Diet

The science that will provide the optimum diet for every American does not yet exist, but it's on its way. The study of "biochemical individuality"—and the determination of personal diets geared to your age, health, genetic heritage, environment, and work conditions—is the ultimate goal of current nutrition research.

"Every individual has a personal blueprint for nutrition," says Dr. Roger Williams, former director of the University of Texas Biomedical Institute. "When diet is not built around that blueprint, genetotropic, or food-related, diseases occur." A healthy body needs proper amounts of about forty chemicals, but no two people have the same requirements. Even two people of the same sex, height, weight, and age, says Williams, can show tenfold differences in basal metabolism (or food-burning) rates. Hence, no single diet or FDA vitamin recommendation can completely satisfy everyone's needs. This is particularly evident from "individuality factors" described by recent nutrition research.

• Nutritionists have discovered variations of a hundredfold and more in the amount of three major intestinal enzymes — lactase, sucrase, and maltase — that break down carbohydrates during digestion. Thus, a diet that provides energy for a husband may make his wife fat.

• A university study of healthy men showed that their calcium requirements varied more than fourfold, from 220 to 1018 milligrams a day. A similar study found that the efficiency with which healthy people break down vital amino acids that help rebuild body cells varies up to sevenfold. Among sick people the variation can be enormous.

• At the Texas Biomedical Institute Dr. Williams discovered that healthy young men who were "knowledgeable about nutrition," and whose diets seemed to be adequate, actually were significantly deficient in vitamin B6. "It is important to realize," he stresses, "that a deficiency existed even in people with an understanding of nutrition who felt that their diet was balanced."

• Nutritionists are also learning that a surprising number of people have "hidden" allergies to such common foods as milk, wheat, eggs, yeast, coffee, chocolate, strawberries. (The list grows longer each year.) A major health problem arises when you become addicted to precisely those foods to which you are allergic. The reason for the addiction: those foods give you a "high." But it's temporary and is always followed by a sharp low. Your body struggles to neutralize a substance that was originally a stimulant but has turned into a toxin, and you are puzzled by your sudden swings in energy. No one yet knows how many of us suffer unsuspectingly from hidden allergies.

• • •

Your personal diet is coming, though. Computers can already analyze blood samples to chart how your body utilizes food. Soon computers will be able to study a strand of hair to determine whether your body is deficient in important trace minerals; to analyze saliva, gastric, and enzymatic juices to reveal your capacity to break down nutrients; to study urine and fecal matter to find out what your body absorbs and what it discards. Even your chromosomes will be analyzed by a computer for genetic deficiencies. The result will be a personal diet modified yearly — or more frequently if conditions in your life and environment change suddenly. (See *Your Hair Tells All*, p. 61.)

Meanwhile, Dr. Williams offers these dietary recommendations: diversify your diet; avoid refined foods and limit the use of sugar, salt, and alcohol; take advantage of vitamin and mineral supplements; and, most important, cultivate your own body wisdom — that is, become aware of the foods that make you feel sluggish and depressed, those that provide energy, and especially the foods that pick you up only to let you down quickly.

Eating to Grow Smart

Foods have long been known to affect the body, but it's come as a complete surprise to scientists that certain foods influence the brain. In the future your diet may play a major role in improving the way your brain functions. You may be eating particular foods to improve memory or to enhance concentration and learning. Breakfast may be planned to awaken your creative or analytic skills for a high-powered day.

Feelings of hunger and thirst are usually attributed to the stomach, but they are, in fact, moods and urges of the brain. Dr. Richard Wurtman, a neuroendocrinologist at the Massachusetts Institute of Technology, is learning that specific foods affect the brain's production of neurotransmitters, chemicals that carry messages between nerve cells. One substance, choline, found abundantly in egg yolks, soybeans, liver, and other foods rich in lecithin, has already been used to cure the malady tardive dyskinesia, the involuntary twitching of the face, tongue, and limbs that follows the long-term use of antipsychotic drugs by mental patients. The disease is known to be caused by a shortage of the neurotransmitter acetylcholine, and Wurtman has successfully treated patients with large doses of choline in the form of lecithin. The body transforms lecithin and choline into acetylcholine.

If you're healthy, what can choline do for you? Scientists at the National Institute of Mental Health claim that large doses of choline appear to improve short-term memory; for instance, they found that people were better able to recall lists of words after taking choline. A severe shortage of choline in your diet (an unlikely possibility if your diet is even halfway sensible) could interfere with memory and learning. No serious researcher is predicting that choline capsules, or lecithin granules, will increase your I.Q.; at least not yet, since research on the ways in which choline affects memory and learning has just started.

Your Blood-Brain Barrier

Another natural nutrient that feeds your brain is tyrosine. Also an amino acid prevalent in protein foods, it enhances the formation of two neurotransmitters in your brain: dopamine and norepinephrine. Insufficient dopamine in the brain is responsible for Parkinson's disease, and an excess of dopamine is considered to be a biochemical cause of schizophrenia. (See *Rx for Schizophrenia*, p.

118.) In healthy people high levels of norepinephrine have been linked with depression and aggressive behavior. (See *Relief from Anxiety and Aggression*, p. 116.) Norepinephrine is also thought to regulate blood pressure, and MIT scientists have recently demonstrated that tyrosine can lower blood pressure in rats, suggesting a possible new strategy in controlling high blood pressure.

Not only do certain foods raise the level of your brain's neurotransmitters, but Wurtman has evidence that "higher levels of these chemicals actually increase the amplitude of the messages sent to the next cell — with probable consequences for behavior." What consequences? Can consuming large quantities of tyrosine help patients with Parkinson's? Make a violent person docile? At the moment no one knows, but experiments with tyrosine have already begun.

The idea that diet can affect the brain contradicts all previous theories. The brain was considered such a sacrosanct organ that it alone was protected by the blood-brain barrier, which prevented almost anything that worked its way into the blood stream from entering the brain. Only certain drugs, glucose, water, and caffeine were thought to penetrate this barrier. "It is a complete surprise," says Wurtman, "that we've been able to manipulate something as important as a chemical transmitter by administering a nutrient." He has preliminary evidence that nutrient deficiencies may also be linked to such ailments as manic episodes and senile memory loss. The poor diets of many older people could be responsible, in part, for such conditions as forgetfulness, impatience, and senility.

Brain-diet research is in its infancy, but the list of foods capable of penetrating the blood-brain barrier is growing. Lack of nutrients can have dramatic effects on your body, causing scurvy, beriberi, muscle fatigue, brittle bones, and anemia. If your brain is deprived of nutrients, you may suffer an even more morbid spectrum of mental and physical ailments. Neuronutritionists also hope eventually to understand the nature of our food preferences — cultural, social, and economic factors aside. Why do many of us, for example, prefer a chocolate bar to an apple, or steak to chicken? We know that our body demands certain foods, but does our brain also signal its own needs?

Eating to Sleep

What to eat at bedtime to promote drowsiness? Is there a food or drink that can alleviate insomnia?

Scientists have discovered that the nutrient tryptophan crosses through the blood-brain barrier. Tryptophan is an amino acid common in milk, cheese, eggs, meats, and especially tuna fish. Your body breaks down tryptophan and feeds it to your brain in the form of the neurotransmitter serotonin, one of the brain's own tranquilizers.

In 1975 researchers at the Maryland Psychiatric Center prescribed tryptophan in pill form for women insomniacs who normally spent over an hour trying to fall asleep. In a matter of days their tossing time had been cut in half and their overall night's sleep extended by forty-five minutes. More recently, doctors at the Boston State Hospital Sleep Laboratory found that one to four grams of tryptophan not only reduced by half the amount of time it took a person to fall asleep, but, unlike traditional sleeping pills, tryptophan did not alter the normal cycles of sleep and dreaming. "Although tryptophan probably won't be powerful enough to calm someone who is highly anxious or agitated," says Sleep Laboratory director Dr. Ernest Hartmann, "my impression is that it will be helpful to many insomniacs, especially on a short-run basis, and will replace many mild sleeping pills."

The Carbohydrate Cure

The brain-diet connection can be awesomely tricky. Should you, for instance, consume foods high in tryptophan in order to fall asleep? No, answers Richard Wurtman. A few other amino acids in high-protein foods can beat tryptophan to the entry points in the brain capillaries and jam the blood-brain barrier; this prevents tryptophan's absorption and conversion to the tranquilizing serotonin.

A surer method of increasing your brain serotonin, says Wurtman, "is to eat a high-carbohydrate, protein-poor meal. Those foods stimulate insulin, which removes the competing amino acids from the blood and allows the blood tryptophan to reach the brain to produce more serotonin." Whole milk is 42 percent more carbohydrate than protein, and even low-fat, protein-fortified milk contains more carbohydrate than protein. So yes, a glass of milk before bed may help you sleep. So, too, may pure tryptophan tablets. As a mild sedative, tryptophan is no panacea for insomnia, but from a health standpoint it is far safer for your body than barbiturates and tranquilizers.

Eating for Better Mental Health

Megavitamin therapy (or orthomolecular medicine, as it's technically called) may never live up to the miraculous claims made by its pioneers in the 1950s. However, it is steadily gaining respectability and creating new medical breakthroughs. Vitamins may one day be used not only to cure certain mental illnesses, but also to prevent them.

In 1968 Linus Pauling, the Nobel laureate chemist, advocated massive doses of vitamin C to cure the common cold, and overnight the ten-year-old, quietly blooming field of megavitamin therapy suddenly attracted the public's attention. Laymen and physicians learned that for years practitioners of megavitamin therapy had been treating schizophrenics with large doses of nicotinic acid (vitamin B3) — and reporting success. These reports came under scathing criticism from the American Medical ·Association. Nicotinic acid, said the AMA, is no more effective against schizophrenia than is ascorbic acid in warding off colds. But after a decade of hearings by the Food and Drug Administration and hundreds of new experiments, medical support for megavitamin therapy is suddenly increasing. In April 1978 the *American Journal of Psychiatry* published the results of the first strictly controlled studies, showing that large doses of pyridoxine (vitamin B6) significantly improved the condition of eleven of sixteen autistic children.

Biochemists know that vitamins are active substances like enzymes and hormones (except that your body can't synthesize them), and that vitamins affect cellular metabolism and regulate chemical processes throughout the body. Knowledge about vitamins has been gained largely through deficiency studies, in which animals are fed vitamin-poor diets. It is much more difficult to document what vitamin-rich diets actually achieve, so research with people continues to progress slowly.

The initial suspicion that nicotinic acid might help schizophrenics was voiced in the 1940s. The vitamin was proved to cure pellagra victims not only of their diarrhea and dermatitis, but also the dementia that accompanies the disease. Reports during the following years indicated that megadoses of vitamins, and combinations of vitamins — primarily niacin, ascorbic acid, pyridoxine, pantothenic acid, and vitamin E — could cure autism, hyperactivity, and learning disabilities in children. Since most of these early experiments were performed with small groups of people, the results are open to doubt. New studies, however, are already underway. The United States Department of Agriculture, the Food and Drug Administration, and the Department of Health, Education, and Welfare are competing to see which agency will set the new nutritional policies for the 1980s and 1990s, and which will revise the recommended dietary allowance (RDA) for each vitamin. (The present RDA was formulated in the 1940s.) Some of the most promising current research concerns the effects of vitamins on your physical health.

Eating for Better Physical Health

Vitamin A

Scientists at the National Cancer Institute in Bethesda, Maryland, are working with vitamin A and its synthetic analogs, retinoids. They have found that in animals this vitamin can prevent cancer of the skin, respiratory tract, mammary glands, and bladder. NCI's Dr. Michael Sporn suggests that a diet deficient in natural retinoids enhances our susceptibility to chemical carcinogens. An epidemiological study of more than 8000 men with equivalent smoking habits linked a low dietary intake of vitamin A with a high incidence of lung cancer. "Combined with the animal studies, that's not proof," says Sporn, "but it's certainly suggestive." Synthetic retinoids act like vitamin A, but with much less toxicity from large doses than can occur with heavy doses of vitamin A.

Vitamin C and Colds

Dozens of studies on the effects of vitamin C on the common cold have yielded conflicting results. Some researchers concluded that the vitamin actually prevented colds, and others claimed it lessened the severity of cold symptoms. Yet in other experiments vitamin C proved to be no more valuable in treating colds than a placebo. The largest controlled study, and the most definitive to date, was done by Dr. Terence Anderson at the University of Toronto. Anderson found that if several grams of vitamin C can't cure your cold, it can palliate cold symptoms and shorten the duration of a cold by 30 percent.

Vitamin C and Cancer

Dr. Ewan Cameron, a Scottish physician, has treated 100 patients with advanced cancer by administering ten grams of vitamin C a day. These patients were compared with 1000 patients who received conventional cancer therapies. The patients on vitamin C, claims Cameron, lived an average of four times longer, and thirteen of them (over twenty times the average of the controls) lost all signs of malignancy. But other researchers, though they followed Cameron's prescription, did not achieve his results. In fact, the studies on vitamin C and cancer are every bit as conflicting as those of vitamin C and colds. If vitamin C does benefit some cancer patients, researchers suspect it's because the vitamin increases the body's production of the viral-fighting antibody interferon, which also attacks cancer cells. (See *Interferon*, p. 34.)

Vitamin E

University of California biochemist Dr. Al Tappel is discovering that vitamin E protects the lungs against environmental pollutants. He first demonstrated with animals that vitamin E could prevent lung damage caused by the nitrogen dioxide in smog. Recently, he began tests with humans and is already observing similar beneficial effects from vitamin E. (Evidence on the alleged benefits of vitamin E in treating and preventing heart diseases, however, remains highly conflicting.) Careful not to overstate the claims for vitamins, Tappel says, "Evolution took place under conditions that didn't involve photochemical smog. The world has been changed by man, especially in the last thirty years or so with the tremendous outpouring of new chemicals. One could question, therefore, whether the nutrient levels man accommodated to are optimized for him at this moment."

. . .

Orthomolecular medicine maintains that many diseases are caused by chemical imbalances in the brain and body. Vitamins, natural constituents, fortify and enhance our body's own protective mechanisms. Thus, the philosophy of orthomolecular medicine is the same as that of the new field of immunotherapy — that with a little natural help, our bodies can, in many instances, heal themselves. Biochemists, incidentally, believe that there are probably vitamins waiting to be identified.

"Vitamin" B15

Is B15 a vitamin? Probably not, according to Food and Drug Administration scientists. No B15–deficiency disease has yet been identified — the sure test of a vitamin. And there are no U.S. studies to back the claims that B15 (pangamic acid) fights fatigue or cures addictions. In 1978 the FDA seized quantitites of the substance from health-food stores and is attempting to gain control over B15 by arguing that it is a food additive. Though B15 may have failed the test for a vitamin, it appears to be more substantial than a placebo. Glenn Shue, an FDA nutritionist who surveyed the extensive Soviet studies on B15 dating back to 1965, says, "B-15 seems to have a very real effect. I am convinced of that from reading the literature. But I don't think it represents, as some have maintained, a vitamin. However, there seems to be evidence that it would be useful as a drug for certain conditions where the body is not able to get enough oxygen."

At present, animal studies are being conducted at several American universities in an attempt to duplicate the Soviet findings. But most researchers agree that what sells in health-food stores as B15 is seldom high-quality (or even real) pangamic acid, and that any benefits reported are largely psychological.

• • •

The real breakthroughs in orthomolecular medicine have yet to come. Despite advances in biochemistry, no one knows how vitamins influence our body and brain, or whether vitamins really bolster our immunological system, and if so, how much. Since cancer, heart disease — and many mental illnesses — take years to develop, they are ideally suited to preventive measures administered in the early stages. There is growing belief that at least several of those measures will originate in medically prescribed vitamin therapy.

A Safe Sweetener

Sweeter than sugar, harmless to teeth, and acceptable to diabetics. These are the claims advanced for a new sweetener that could soon replace cyclamates, saccharin, and even sugar.

The new substance, called NHDC (neohesperidin dihydrochalcone), is derived from grapefruits and oranges. Not wanting to release a chemical for public consumption that may later be indicted as a carcinogen, industry and government scientists have tested NHDC on rats and dogs for five years; to date, animals force-fed enormous quantities have shown no ill effects, and according to dental tests NHDC does not contribute to tooth decay.

Since NHDC is more than 1000 times sweeter than sugar, less of it would be needed to sweeten beverages, whose caloric content would be proportionately lower. Scientists at the Agriculture Department's Fruit and Vegetable Chemistry Division say that NHDC's sensation of sweetness is slow in coming and long in duration. The fact that the sweetness lingers on your taste buds makes it ideal in such products as chewing gum, candies, soft drinks, mouth washes, and toothpastes. If all this sounds too good to be true, NHDC does have one disadvantage: it leaves an aftertaste that some scientists liken to licorice and others to menthol. You'll be able to decide for yourself, since NHDC is to be licensed for commercial use in the early 1980s.

Your Caffeine Addiction

Is caffeine a lethal drug or an ingredient in a harmless, stimulating drink? Is it true that a pregnant woman who drinks eight cups of coffee a day may have a baby who isn't completely normal?

Tens of thousands of years ago man first stumbled on caffeine's stimulating effects. But never have more people consumed it in so many forms and in such large quantities as today. Since coffee, tea, and caffeine-laced colas are predominant beverages internationally, the questions concerning the safety of caffeine have scientists worried — and divided. On one thing they do agree: if caffeine were introduced today as a new product, it would be available only by prescription. A vast amount of new research is in progress to determine the effects of caffeine on the human brain, body, and fetus. The evidence thus far includes these facts and warnings:

• A cup of tea or coffee contains between 100 to 150 milligrams of caffeine; cola drinks 35 to 55 milligrams a bottle; and 20 milligrams are in a one-ounce chocolate bar.

• Caffeine can kill. Animals fed massive doses have gone into cardiac arrest. In man, the lethal dose is about 10,000 milligrams — or ninety cups of coffee consumed within about two hours.

• The half-life of caffeine in your body varies from three to five hours. There is no accumulation of the drug; it disappears from your body almost completely overnight.

• Caffeine can be addictive, and abrupt withdrawal results in severe headaches and shaking. Its addictive properties have been clearly demonstrated in animals: once given a taste of caffeine

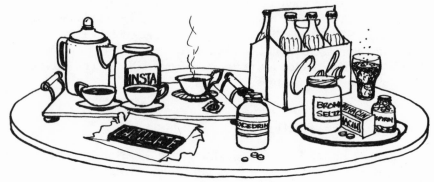

Brewed coffee 100-150 mg.
Instant coffee 85-95 mg.
Tea 60-75 mg. Cola drink 40-80 mg.

Chocolate bar   Exedrin   Bromo Seltzer
1oz   20 mg.   tablet   66 mg.   Anacin
                                          Aspirin
                                          tablet   32 mg.

Caffeine Content

Caffeine exists in many products. Although apparently harmless in small quantities, caffeine can kill; the lethal dose for humans is ten grams — or 100 cups of coffee — consumed in about four hours. A pregnant woman who drinks 8 cups of coffee a day may have a baby who isn't completely normal. If caffeine were to be introduced as a new drug today, you would probably need a prescription to obtain it.

added to their water, animals prefer caffeinated water to unadulterated water.

• If you consume large quantities of caffeine regularly, it's easy to develop a tolerance for it — which means you then have to take more to get a lift.

• Contrary to popular belief, caffeine strongly *increases* the impaired performance caused by alcohol. There is no proof that caffeine, by itself, has a sobering influence.

• In bacteria, fungi, and algae, caffeine is a potent cause of genetic mutations. It also inhibits the self-repair mechanisms of cells that act to minimize the damage to DNA caused by ultraviolet sunlight.

• In mice, rats, man, and other mammals, however, all attempts to demonstrate caffeine as a mutagen have so far failed — although experiments show that male rats lose their ability to produce sperm and suffer atrophy of the reproductive organs when fed large quantities of caffeine. Nor has the drug been positively linked with heart disease or cancer. Judging by current studies, higher forms of life metabolize caffeine much more easily than lower organisms — and this may account for the deleterious effects of caffeine on lower forms of life.

• Caffeine consumed by pregnant women may have adverse effects on their babies. Dr. Ann Streissguth of the University of Washington has produced preliminary findings that show babies born to women who drink eight or more cups of coffee a day have less muscle tone and are less active than normal babies. The results of studies to determine whether mothers who consume heavy amounts of caffeine suffer more spontaneous abortions are due in 1981, and Dr. Streissguth's follow-up report on the babies she is studying should be published in 1982. The final verdict is not in, but it appears that caffeine — only when consumed in moderate amounts — is probably one of life's harmless pleasures.

Wine for the Flu

Most people would be grateful for a sound medical excuse to drink alcohol. And one may be forthcoming. Viruses, which seem immune to most modern drugs, succumb to grape juice and wine.

Scientists at Canada's Health and Welfare Department have been experimenting with the old wives' tale that wine combats the common cold. In 1977 they added red and white wine and grape juice to virus-cell cultures. Herpes simplex virus, echo and Coxsackie viruses, were all rendered inactive by the beverages; polio virus was the most severely affected. Purple grape juice proved the most effective killer, followed by a lethal Burgundy, then a moderately fatal Chablis. (No rosé was tested.) Does this mean grape juice and wine also kill viruses in your body?

Scientists at the University of Wisconsin are attempting to answer that question. They raised baby pigs — whose digestive system closely resembles ours — on a human diet, then killed the piglets and mixed their gastrointestinal fluids with viruses that had been inactivated by grape juice. The results were disappointing: within an hour, between 50 to 75 percent of the virus particles had been resurrected. When they mixed inactivated viruses with human blood serum, 94 percent of the virus particles came to life.

The reason for the reversal remains a mystery, but grape juice does have some curative effect. The researchers believe that small molecules from grapes — perhaps phenols — bind to the surface of a virus and prevent it from invading healthy cells. Phenol compounds exist largely in the skin of grapes and only sparsely in the pulp. Depending on the manufacturing process, some juices and wines contain more phenols than others. If the phenol hypothesis turns out to be accurate, a more effective flu remedy might be to eat grapes rather than drink their juice. While scientists are trying to unravel the biochemistry between grapes and viruses, the next time you get the flu, play it safe and down grapes, grape juice, and wine. It certainly will do you no harm.

3

Cancer Breakthroughs:
New Drugs, Tests, Treatments
– and Maybe a Cure

Cancer has long been viewed as an attack by a foreign invader on a healthy but helpless body, and cancer cells were thought to be hopelessly errant cells that had to be killed. Now there is an auspicious new way to view cancer, as a breakdown in the biochemical signals in our genes that can be reversed.

According to this new theory, carcinogenic chemicals and viruses are only *potential* troublemakers. Whether they actually cause trouble depends largely on your state of mental and physical fitness. This philosophy is opening up fresh areas of research that are already showing us that (1) the body is naturally immune to cancer throughout most of its life, except for infancy and old age, the times when our immune system is weakest; (2) at any age stress weakens our immune system, exposing it to the effects of both environmental carcinogens and abnormalities that have been latent in our genes since birth; and (3) our body can bolster itself against cancer by a new treatment called immunotherapy. In our lifetime we are going to witness many breakthroughs in the battle against cancer — and maybe even the ultimate breakthrough, a cure. Here is what you can expect.

Your Low-Risk Cancer Diet

The manner in which we eat and cook our food may contribute to 60 percent of the nation's cancer deaths. This recent alarming statistic from the National Cancer Institute should lead you to alter your diet and the ways in which you prepare foods for the rest of your life. Unfortunately, for several reasons a nationwide change in diet may not occur for at least another decade.

Although there is much evidence suggesting that certain foods increase the risk of cancer, shamefully little research has been done in the field of nutrition. As of 1979, a scant 1 percent of the applications for research grants received by the NCI proposed to study the cancer-diet connection. The reason, asserts Arthur Upton, director of the NCI, is that nutrition research takes decades; a definitive study tracing the link between nutrition and breast cancer, for example, might involve placing a thousand baby girls on a carefully controlled diet and then following them for seventy years to determine the effect of diet. A single project could occupy a scientist's entire professional career. Consequently, the diet-cancer link is being forged slowly, largely from animal experiments and retrospective population studies. Some suggestions for a low-risk cancer diet have already begun to emerge, and throughout the 1980s additional recommendations will be announced almost yearly. Here is what is known — or suspected — concerning the connection between diet and cancer.

Fats and Men

Diets high in fats (especially meat fats) result in the production of bile acids, produced by the liver to digest fat. Excessive bile acids in the stool may cause cancer of the colon and rectum in men. Evidence for this is strong but not yet conclusive. In a new study, British researchers recently collected and stored stool samples from 7500 adults. Their health and dietary habits will be followed for five years, and those who develop colon cancer will have their stools analyzed for excessive bile acids. Researchers have reason to suspect that perhaps only 10 percent of the population is particularly vulnerable to colon cancer from high-fat diets. By 1985 they hope to know why and to have proof of the fat–colon cancer connection.

Fats and Women

Breast cancer shows a strong link to diet. In countries where women consume high levels of fat and animal protein, there is a higher incidence of breast cancer. Scientists believe that a high-fat diet may increase the amount of the female hormone prolactin in the blood, promoting mammary tumors.

Fiber

If fat contributes to colon cancer, a high-fiber diet may help counteract fat's deleterious effects. Fiber makes stools firm, and that quickens their transit through the bowels. So there's less time for carcinogens to linger on bowel walls, where they can cause mutations that make cells malignant. According to the medical journal *The Lancet*, the foods that produce the most robust bowel movements and hasten the passage of stools through the large intestine are, in order of effectiveness, bran, cabbage, carrots, and apples. In general, first cereals, then vegetables, then fruits.

Vitamin C

The large amounts of vitamin C in the American diet may explain why there is a lower incidence of stomach cancer in the United States than in countries like Japan, where diets are low in vitamin C. Japanese who migrate to America and switch to a diet containing less rice and other starches and more fruits and vegetables experience a reduced risk of stomach cancer. Researchers at the American Health Foundation suspect that the vitamin C in juices, fruits, and vegetables protects the stomach against the conversion of nitrites into carcinogenic nitrosamines. (See *Eating for Better Physical Health*, p. 18.)

Selenium

The element selenium, which is found in certain foods, also seems to help reduce the risk of cancer. According to the National Cancer Institute, populations throughout the world that subsist on diets high in selenium-rich foods have a significantly lower incidence of cancer of the colon, stomach, lungs, and bladder. In fact, for some unknown reason, selenium seems to protect against almost all types of cancer. "It is clear that selenium is an important element in the whole story of cancer in general," says NCI's Dr. Pietro Gullino. Foods rich in selenium are fish, liver, kidney, onions, garlic, mushrooms, eggs, and wheat cereals.

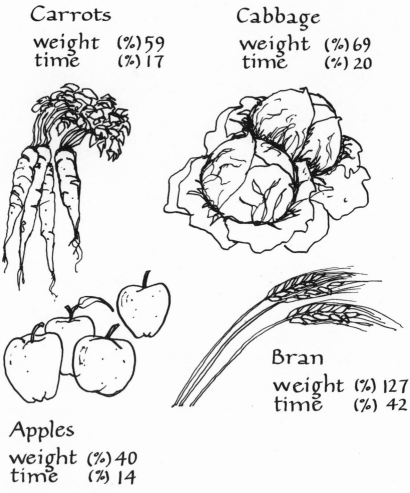

Carrots
weight (%) 59
time (%) 17

Cabbage
weight (%) 69
time (%) 20

Bran
weight (%) 127
time (%) 42

Apples
weight (%) 40
time (%) 14

Fabulous Fiber Foods

The fiber content of certain foods increases fecal weight and shortens the time that residue remains in the large intestine. Firmer stools move more quickly through the intestine and may reduce the risk of colon cancer. Bran, for example, is the best dietary source of fiber because it increases fecal weight 127 percent and shortens the time stools are held in the large intestine by 42 percent. The next best foods are cabbage, carrots, then apples.

Cholesterol

Although a high-cholesterol diet may clog your arteries and increase your risk of a heart attack, the cholesterol produced by your own body may safeguard you from all kinds of cancer. It now appears that endogenous cholesterol may be the means that the fighters in your immune system — the T cells — need to destroy tumors; without it they may be helpless against malignancy, as well as bacterial and viral infections. The scientists at the Jackson Laboratory in Maine and the Swiss Institute of Experimental Cancer Research who made this recent discovery still aren't sure just how endogenous cholesterol fortifies T cells. As a result of their work, a simple blood test that reveals your body's cholesterol production may one day enable your doctor to estimate the natural strength of your immune system and your native ability to combat not only cancer but other diseases as well.

Early-Detection Tests

A cure for cancer may be decades away, but new tests to detect certain kinds of cancer in its early stages will be appearing almost yearly during the 1980s. Through the early detection of malignant cells, the tests could save countless lives. Here are two of the many tests you can expect.

For Women: A Skin Test for Breast Cancer

For women over thirty-five, breast tumors are the leading cause of cancer death. Scientists at Evanston Hospital in Illinois have discovered that women with breast tumors produce a chemical called "active" T-antigen in their mammary tissues and blood, but healthy women produce an "inactive" version of the compound. When the Illinois doctors injected active T-antigen under the skin of 100 women who were suspected of having breast cancer, all but two of those who developed inflamed red blotches at the site of the injection turned out to have breast cancer when biopsies were performed. And only three women who had breast cancer failed to show an allergic reaction to the T-antigen. If researchers at the Sloan-Kettering Institute for Cancer Research in New York are successful in their attempt to duplicate the Illinois results, by the mid 1980s women may be able to have a simple early screening for breast cancer without the radiation risk posed by X rays.

For Men: A Blood Test for Prostate Cancer

Of the 70,000 American men who develop cancer of the prostate gland each year, more than a third die because the cancer was not detected early enough: many men simply refuse to submit to the rectal examination by which a doctor can easily feel a developing tumor. Soon, however, a man may need only to donate a little blood to know if his prostate is becoming cancerous.

For forty years doctors have attempted to use blood tests to detect the minute traces of the enzyme phosphatase, which signals prostate cancer. But the tests have seldom been successful, because none was adequately sensitive to detect the enzyme. Now, through the use of a technique called radioimmunoassay, for which the 1977 Nobel prize in medicine was awarded, scientists in the United States and England can detect a billionth of a gram of phosphatase in a man's blood. Clinical tests in both countries show that the new procedures can detect prostate cancer in its first stage in at least 30 percent of the men who have it; and the blood test quickly becomes more accurate as the condition progresses. Scientists are working to refine the technique further, and if they succeed, a blood test for prostate cancer could be a routine medical procedure by 1983.

Your Doctor's New Anticancer Drugs

A new line — and a new generation — of anticancer drugs is on the way. Some will relieve pain, others will halt the spread of malignancy, and a few will be designed by computers to kill off cancer cells selectively, leaving healthy cells unharmed. Here's a representative look at the breakthroughs you can expect.

The Killer Compound

Scientists at the University of California School of Medicine at San Francisco knew what they wanted an anticancer drug to be: a chemical that latched onto cancer cells not for a few seconds, as most drugs do, but for minutes at a time, delivering its lethal punch. In 1978 they fed a computer all their information about the biology of cancer and the human immunological system. The computer drew on a screen in three-dimensional perspective the molecular structure of possible potent drugs. It performed a commendable job, for when the scientists selected one of the most lethal-looking of the drugs and synthesized it, they discovered that a single dose killed hundreds of millions of cancer cells in mice. They named the drug azetomicin, and it is probably the most potent anticancer drug ever produced — mainly because it clings to cancer cells, destroying their chemical structure, for an amazing twenty-six minutes, a marathon record among anti-cancer drugs. Azetomicin will be tested on cancer patients during the early 1980s. If it is anywhere near as effective as scientists hope it will be, we shall soon be treated by a whole generation of powerful computer-designed drugs, each tailored for one of the many different kinds of malignant cells in which cancer masquerades.

The Normalizing Compound

Dr. Daniel Dexter of the Brown University Medical School is one of the major proponents of the new notion that cancer is not a permanent condition of a cell, but a temporary state that can be reversed with the aid of the proper drug. After years of research, Dexter, working with Dr. Roger Williams, now thinks he's found such a drug: DMF (dimethyl formamide). He discovered that when it is added to cultures of malignant human colon cells, DMF returned them to a healthy state. Encouraged by this observation, he tried the drug on human cancerous breast and muscle tumors and achieved the same results. Finally, he injected DMF into mice on which human tumors had been grafted, and within ten days the tumors were either dead or in the process of dying. Dr. Dexter intends to repeat his tests on a larger population of animals. It may be several years before clinical tests include cancer patients, but even at this early stage of research he thinks he may have some inkling as to how DMF works: cancer cells are immature, sort of children frozen in time at prepuberty; DMF somehow "educates" these cells and forces them to mature to carry out their life function.

Pot

So agonizing are the side effects of chemotherapy that many patients choose to count on luck for a remission or cure rather than undergo treatment. Compazine has proven to be only moderately effective in relieving chemotherapy's intense symptoms of nausea and vomiting. THC, the hallucinogenic ingredient in marijuana, seems more effective, but THC research has progressed slowly because of the drug's illegal status and because several critics object to its addicting nature and the euphoria it produces.

A promising new drug developed by Eli Lilly and Company is Nabilone. It appears to be every bit as potent as THC in combating nausea and vomiting, but it doesn't induce euphoria. Lilly scientists had originally set out to develop a new tranquilizer, but found that their new drug was better as an antiemetic. After three years of clinical tests on cancer patients, the scientists believe that Nabilone is no panacea for all the symptoms of chemotherapy, but for many people it is remarkably beneficial. Its most common side effects are drowsiness, a parched mouth, and minor loss of coordination. Lilly scientists expect the drug to be available by 1981.

Heroin

More than half of all cancer patients suffer agonizing pain in the final stages of their illness. Doctors at Sloan-Kettering have been testing morphine on terminal cancer patients and claim that it works in 95 percent of the cases. They extended their experimental program in 1978 to include heroin and are already finding that it appears to be a better painkiller than morphine. Since heroin is a more powerful drug, it can be given in smaller doses and administered more frequently, thereby providing longer periods of pain relief. They expect to complete their present tests with heroin in the early 1980s, and believe that pain in terminal cancer patients may soon be treated with narcotics.

A Miracle Compound?

Will Laetrile, the controversial apricot-pit extract, contribute a major breakthrough in cancer therapy? Over a dozen states have legalized the manufacture, sale, and use of Laetrile, and the furor surrounding the drug prompted the American Cancer Society in 1978 to sponsor its own clinical tests on several hundred terminal patients. So conflicting have been Laetrile test results that the staffs of several top laboratories, Sloan-Kettering for one, are split (if not down the middle) over the merits of the drug. The ACS hopes to separate fact from fiction when the final results of their tests are completed and analyzed in the early 1980s. Should Laetrile prove to be the least bit effective, pharmaceutical companies are geared up for mass production. However, even if the ACS tests are flatly negative, many scientists fear that a significant portion of the population, hungry for a cancer cure, will cling to the false hope of Laetrile's curative power.

A Personal Treatment Plan

Anticancer drugs, especially new ones, can be tricky to administer, for doctors can't always predict a patient's reaction to a certain drug. Sometimes a patient must experiment with several powerful drugs that can have ghastly side effects before the doctor discovers which drug kills the cancer cells. Researchers at the University of Arizona Cancer Center, however, are on the brink of a breakthrough that may soon put an end to this trial-and-error approach to drug treatment. They have learned how to grow a patient's cancer cells in a Petri dish so that the cells respond to anticancer drugs the same way they react in the patient's body.

The scientists extracted malignant ovarian tissue from nine women, and cancerous bone marrow from nine other patients, and treated these samples with various concentrations of several anticancer drugs, then cultured the tissues with a special new treatment in Petri dishes. When the same drugs were tested directly on the patients, the scientists found that a drug that killed a patient's cultured cancer cells was as effective in the patient, and when the drug had no effect in the Petri dish it did not help the patient. This experiment also confirmed the frustrating, unexplainable fact that, though several patients may suffer from the exact kind of cancer, their cells in culture can show up to a thirtyfold variation in response to the same drug — a difference the patients themselves also demonstrate.

Much more work needs to be done before the special culture technique can be applied to the various kinds of cancer. But the Arizona researchers envision a day in the not-too-distant future — perhaps the late 1980s — when doctors won't have to use people as guinea pigs for new anticancer drugs. Even more promising, the culture technique will eventually enable a doctor to plan a highly effective, personalized treatment for a patient — before a single drug is prescribed for the patient.

Your Body's Own Anticancer Drugs

Since the time of Louis Pasteur, doctors have fought disease with drugs derived from microbes, plants, and compounds concocted in laboratories. In the near future, however, a doctor will help you rally your immune system so that your body will fight its own battles with its own arsenal of killer drugs. This original approach to medicine, immunotherapy, is already showing great promise in combating cancer.

Doctors have often observed with a mixture of awe and perplexity that some cancer patients develop a resistance to cancer after their body successfully fights off an unrelated infection. In 1972, researchers at the Albany Medical Center in New York examined the records of patients who had undergone surgery for lung cancer and found that patients who had been stricken with lung infections after surgery survived much longer than patients who had remained healthy after surgery. Later, Canadian scientists observed that children vaccinated against a form of tuberculosis were less likely to develop leukemia than children who had not been immunized. These and other studies have convinced doctors that when the immune system is stimulated to fight a bacterial, viral, or even a chemical invader, it often will attack and kill cancer cells as well.

Transfer Factor

In healthy people immune-system cells called lymphocytes kill off cancer cells daily before they root and colonize. Apparently when a person develops cancer, his or her immune defenses are "sleeping" on the job. Scientists at the University of Michigan have found at least one chemical in the blood that can "awaken" those immune defenses. They call this substance the transfer factor, because they discovered that when blood taken from someone who has successfully fought cancer is injected into a cancer patient, the new blood helps the patient fight his or her own cancer. The scientists soon hope to isolate the exact chemicals that make up the transfer factor, which is now commonly referred to as "an immunological phenomenon in search of a molecule." Once isolated, the compound could possibly be synthesized by biochemists to provide wide-scale effective treatment for cancer. Scientists believe there may be other transfer factors for different diseases, and that one day these, too, can be prescribed as natural drugs to boost our immune defenses that have been weakened by stress, fatigue, environmental pollutants, or simply old age.

Interferon

Another of our natural body ingredients that appears to fight cancer is interferon, an extract from white blood cells. When it was first discovered, in 1957, interferon was used to kill viruses in animals. Only within the last few years have scientists learned that it can prevent flu, colds, and halt the spread of herpes infections. More recently, doctors have begun to administer interferon to cancer patients. The results have been encouraging. Dr. Jordan Gutterman of Houston's M. D. Anderson Hospital and Tumor Institute has used interferon to shrink advanced breast cancer in several women, and Dr. Thomas Merigan of Stanford University has found that interferon can help patients with cancer of the lymphatic system. Because it's a natural body substance, interferon seems to produce none of the debilitating side effects that accompany most other anticancer drugs.

Scientists believe that invading viruses trigger our body cells to manufacture interferon, which then travels throughout our bodies to combat infections. But evidently it's not interferon's antiviral properties that are responsible for destroying cancer cells (as one might suspect, since some forms of cancer may be caused by viruses). Instead, says Dr. Merigan, interferon seems to fortify a person's immune defenses, which in turn destroy malignancy. "We think that our studies clearly demonstrate activity of human interferon against a human tumor."

Research with interferon is progressing slowly, because the substance is scarce and expensive to extract from white blood cells; a millionth of an ounce costs about $1500. The American Cancer Society has purchased $2 million worth of interferon from Finland, the main producer of the substance, for clinical tests to be conducted in the early 1980s. Gutterman and Merigan will receive batches of this interferon so that they can continue their research. The rest will be divided among several major institutions: the Sloan-Kettering Institute for Cancer Research (for tests on patients with lung and bladder cancer); Roswell Park Memorial Institute in Buffalo, New York (for breast and bladder cancer tests); and Columbia University's College of Physicians and Surgeons (for tests on several common forms of cancer).

Researchers are careful not to overstate the potential benefits of interferon until clinical tests are completed in the mid 1980s. However, if interferon proves to be effective in combating cancer — and if it can be synthesized and mass produced — it would be possible in the future for doctors to prescribe interferon routinely for the elderly, reducing the danger of cancer. It could also be administered over a lifetime to children whose family history shows that they may have a propensity toward cancer.

Chemicals You Should Fear

Although nutritionists claim that as much as 60 percent of all cancers are caused by diet, environmental scientists argue that about 80 percent of human cancers are triggered by natural and artificial elements in our environment — nitrites, asbestos, tars, soot, saccharine, PVC, PCB, DES, DDT, estrogen, and dyes for hair, clothes, and cosmetics — a list of about 3000 compounds — to which, in all fairness, we must add natural and manmade alpha particles, beta particles, gamma rays, and cosmic-ray showers. Whether or not environmentalists have exaggerated their case, given an estimated 100,000 chemicals currently in use in the Western industrial world, and thousands of new chemicals concocted in laboratories each year, it is reassuring to know that there is a concerted drive to develop quick, reliable tests to identify those chemicals which are carcinogens.

The most promising tests all measure the effects of chemicals on special strains of micro-organisms. For instance, the Ames Test for mutagenicity (cell changes that *may* lead to cancer) and carcinogenicity (cell changes that *do* lead to cancer) identifies about 90 percent of the chemicals known to cause cancer, and gives a seal of approval to 85 percent of the chemicals we know are harmless. At present, it's the most accurate method of screening new chemicals. However, at Britain's Imperial Chemical Industries, Ltd., scientists are working on a micro-organism test procedure they hope will surpass the Ames Test in both speed and accuracy. They claim it could gain widespread acceptance by the mid 1980s.

By then, however, Dr. Bruce Ames expects to have honed his own test (already used by several chemical companies) so that it's faster to conduct and 95 percent reliable. As a result of both the improved Ames Test and the British test there should be a sharp decline in the number of unsafe chemicals introduced into the environment. Companies will be able to screen new chemicals quickly and inexpensively and discard them if tests show they're potentially dangerous. This routine testing not only would save millions of dollars spent for manufacturing a chemical that proves to be carcinogenic, but also would save millions of lives.

Firecracker Therapy

Ever since Marie Curie discovered radium, doctors have been treating cancer patients with various kinds of radiation — X rays and gamma rays (which are pure energy), and subatomic chunks of alpha and beta particles and neutrons. But an exotic particle — the pion — that behaves like the most splendid star-burst firecracker may just prove to be the most effective weapon against cancer. At least, this is the hope of physicists and physicians who are beginning a series of the most expensive, tediously precise radiotherapy tests ever conducted to treat cancer patients.

First discovered in the late 1940s, pions are particles that provide the glue holding together the nuclei of atoms. Pions are released in copious streams when nuclei are bombarded with other subatomic particles, and pions can be manipulated by magnetic fields to form thin, accurately aimed beams to treat tumors. A beam of pions can be driven to a precise depth within a patient's body. Once they reach the site of a tumor, the pions explode to form "pion stars" — showers of nuclear debris that fly in every direction, causing lethal damage to diseased tissue over a very short distance. If carefully aimed at their target, pion beams do amazingly little harm to healthy tissue. Thus, pions have a major advantage over other forms of radiation therapy like X rays and gamma rays, which can scatter widely on entering a patient's body, often killing more healthy than cancerous tissue. Though alpha, beta, and neutron particles scatter less, they, too, destroy healthy cells.

The first tests using pion beams on cancer patients were conducted by Dr. Morton Kligerman of the University of New Mexico in the late 1970s, with highly encouraging results. In some of Dr. Kligerman's sixty-seven patients, tumors shrank and stayed in remission for almost a year, and virtually all his patients experienced less of the vomiting and diarrhea that accompanies conventional radiotherapy. From those tests Dr. Kligerman concluded that pions appear to be almost 40 percent more effective than X rays in killing cancer cells.

While Dr. Kligerman continues his research, clinical tests with pion therapy will be conducted during the early 1980s at a research center near Zürich, Switzerland, and in Vancouver, Canada, where large particle accelerators are available to produce pions. In most of the experiments doctors will focus on treating patients with deep-seated tumors of the brain, head, neck, lungs, abdomen, and bladder. The tests are expected to take at least five years to complete. Besides the usual complexities of trying to evaluate a new, sophisticated technology, doctors — because of the precision of pion beams — must design fresh procedures for pinpointing tumors and for orienting and immobilizing patients

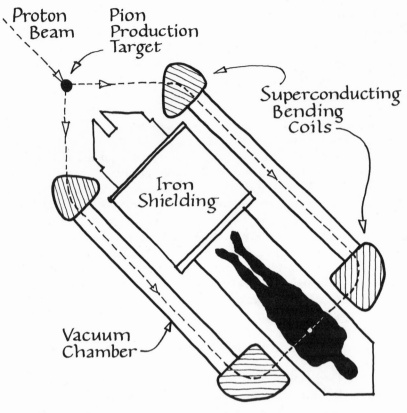

Pion Cancer Therapy

Beams composed of elementary particles called pions (which are 270 times smaller than electrons) are deflected around a huge iron shield and precisely aimed at a patient by superconducting coils. On entering the body, pions go directly to their target, a tumor, and explode within the diseased tissue.

so that the beams strike malignant growths on target. Dr. Kligerman and his colleagues think that the number of patients who now report tumor regression from conventional radiotherapy for a period of five years — the so-called five-year cure — may, with pion therapy, experience a 200-to-300 percent increase in the period of remission.

4

Heart Breakthroughs:
Keep Your Heart Young, Healthy, and Alive

Death from heart disease has been decreasing steadily since 1968, and several factors are responsible: earlier detection of potential heart trouble, new drugs to lower high blood pressure and open clogged arteries, improved dietary habits, and an increase in the number of people who exercise. Nevertheless, heart disease still causes more deaths each year than any other illness, and attempts to reduce the danger of heart attacks will take many interesting new turns during the decade ahead. In this section we'll look at some of the ingenious new drugs, therapies, and dietary habits that may, by the end of the decade, bounce heart disease from the number one spot on the list of America's most deadly diseases.

A New Cholesterol Test

The amount of cholesterol in your blood may have a minimal effect on your health and even less effect on coronary artery disease. Further, present blood tests that measure serum cholesterol levels may prove useless, to be replaced in a few years by more relevant procedures.

Though this contradicts a decade of medical warnings concerning cholesterol, more and more doctors are adopting this philosophy. And with good reason. The real heart-disease culprits appear

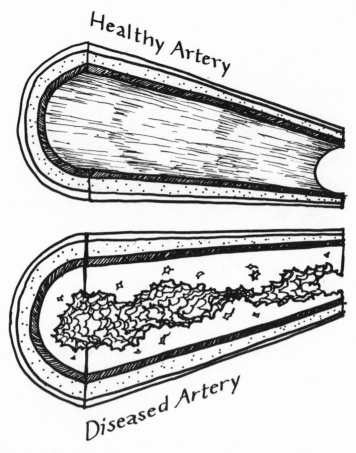

Healthy Artery

Diseased Artery

Cholesterol Clogging

Atherosclerosis is the buildup of cholesterol on arterial walls. However, the amount of cholesterol in the blood may have a minimal effect on the development of coronary-artery disease. A more significant measure of heart-attack risk may be the ratio of "good" to "bad" protein molecules that transport cholesterol throughout the body.

to be protein molecules that transport cholesterol throughout the body. And the ratio of these "good" to "bad" carriers may be what actually determines your risk of heart disease.

Cholesterol, whether it is derived from food or manufactured by the body, travels through your system on the back of molecules called lipoproteins. These come in two basic varieties: the "good" high-density lipoproteins (HDL), which rush cholesterol to the metabolic pathway and on to excretion; and the "bad" low-density lipoproteins (LDL), which deposit cholesterol-like sludge on arterial walls. Rats are resistant to atherosclerosis (the accumulation of cholesterol on arterial walls); they are blessed with primarily HDL. Pigs, dogs, apes, and people who suffer from atherosclerosis are plagued with mostly LDL. Epidemiological studies also record that those of us lucky enough to have more HDL than LDL run much less risk of heart disease.

Danger Foods

For a while it was popularly thought that genes and exercise more than diet largely determined a person's HDL:LDL ratio. Some doctors even scoffed at the notion that a diet high in eggs, the most concentrated form of cholesterol in the human diet, contributed to a higher incidence of heart disease. Research at the National Heart, Lung, and Blood Institute, however, is changing that picture. Eggs and other foods loaded with cholesterol may end up on a "Very High Danger" list. It now seems that the beneficial cholesterol carrier HDL also occurs in an unhealthy variety, which researchers have labeled HDL-c. It acts like LDL. Even more astonishing, people who eat eggs actually begin producing HDL-c. This recent discovery could explain a fact that has long puzzled doctors: a high-cholesterol diet can clog the arteries of people with low blood-cholesterol levels.

In the NHLBI study, healthy men and women ate four to six eggs a day for a month. All developed increases in HDL-c — even those whose total blood-cholesterol levels did not increase! Do other high-cholesterol foods produce HDL-c? They do in dogs, swine, rats, rabbits, and monkeys, and that is almost a guarantee that human tests now in progress will yield similar results. "The really important question," says Dr. Robert Mahley, who headed the study, "may be not how much cholesterol is in the blood but what type of lipoprotein carries it around."

Since most doctors measure only blood-cholesterol levels, they could be missing early-warning signs of atherosclerosis in their patients. Tests exist to measure the lipoprotein ratios, but they cost almost twice as much as the standard serum cholesterol test, so they're performed only on request. In a few years, however, lipoprotein tests may be deemed so essential in determining our physical fitness that they may well become a standard part of our medical checkup.

Cholesterol Cleaner

It pours like vegetable oil and spreads like margarine. You can eat it to your heart's delight because it doesn't contain calories. And, most amazing, it removes only the deleterious cholesterol from your body, leaving the good cholesterol unaffected. This miracle product — sucrose polyester (SPE) — which has already been successfully tested at two research centers, is under Food and Drug Administration inspection, and could be commercially available, with a more appetizing name, by 1985.

Sucrose polyester possesses all the culinary qualities of a good vegetable oil, but it's a synthetic, made in the laboratory by reacting sucrose, a sugar, with long-chain fatty acids. Tests on men and women in Ohio and California have shown that SPE eliminates both the cholesterol derived from food and that manufactured by the body. More important, SPE reduces the amount of "bad" LDL-linked cholesterol believed to cause coronary-artery disease, and leaves the "good" HDL-linked cholesterol intact.

Sucrose polyester acts in the intestine by attaching itself only to cholesterol carried by LDL molecules. Its own molecules are so large that they are not absorbed but are excreted whole, taking cholesterol with them. SPE's only side effect seems to be that it interferes with the absorption of vitamins A and E. Doctors believe that people who use SPE will have to include vitamin supplements in their diets. Although SPE appears to be nothing more than vegetable oil, the FDA considers it a drug and therefore must complete its own safety tests before it will allow markets to stock it.

Cholesterol Sponge

If you have inherited a tendency for high blood cholesterol, a low-fat diet cannot guarantee you a low cholesterol level. There are, of course, several drugs your doctor can prescribe to lower your cholesterol count by as much as 25 percent. For some people this reduction is sufficient to transfer them from a high-risk heart-attack category to a low one. For others, though, such drugs have very little effect. In a few years, however, doctors may be able to prescribe one of two drugs — colestipol or nicotinic acid — that could halve the amount of cholesterol in anyone's blood.

These two drugs, which have been tested on people with inherited tendencies toward high cholesterol, look extremely promising. Both drugs act to reduce cholesterol in very direct ways. Nicotinic acid causes your body to produce less low-density lipoprotein (LDL), the apparent cause of cholesterol buildup on artery walls; whereas colestipol acts like a sponge to soak up cholesterol and carry it through the intestine and out of the body.

In tests at the University of California School of Medicine in San Francisco, 90 percent of the patients who took either one of the drugs and maintained a low-fat diet for a year were rewarded when their blood-cholesterol levels returned to normal. More extensive tests with the drugs are underway. If they prove successful, and the drugs receive FDA approval, they could effectively lower the risk of heart attack for thousands of people by the end of the decade.

Home Remedies for Your Heart

Some time during the 1980s it may be solidly proved that the risk of a second heart attack — and maybe a first — can be reduced with the aid of a few aspirins and a little alcohol every day, not, of course, taken together. Several researchers are currently examining this possibility.

Aspirin

As early as the 1950s, anecdotal evidence suggested that the properties of aspirin that prevent blood clotting may lessen the chance of heart attack by facilitating circulation. Recently, several studies have supported, though not yet proved, that earlier suspicion. In an extensive study in 1974, Boston researchers examined the hospital records of more than 8000 patients and determined that those patients taking aspirin regularly were less prone to heart problems. In the hope of establishing a link between aspirin and heart-attack risk, scientists working for the federally funded Aspirin Myocardial Infarction Study are currently monitoring the health of 4500 men and women between the ages of thirty and seventy who have already suffered one heart attack. Some in the group are given three aspirins a day; others get placebos. By observing the incidence of minor and major heart attacks over a period of three years, the scientists hope to establish conclusively whether aspirin can prevent a second attack. If so, scientists will then tackle the even bigger question: Can daily doses of aspirin, taken under a doctor's supervision, improve our chances of avoiding a first heart attack?

Although aspirin may prove to be a simple, inexpensive treatment, or even a preventive measure, for certain heart problems, doctors caution us that no firm link yet exists between aspirin and heart-attack risk, and that heavy doses of aspirin can cause gastrointestinal bleeding and damage the kidneys and liver. What's more, California cardiologists have recently learned that women who take excessive amounts of aspirin during pregnancy may give birth to children plagued with hypertension and the risk of heart failure early in life.

Prevention of Spasms

It's possible that aspirin, as well as other anticoagulant drugs, treat only a symptom of heart disease — blood clotting — rather than the root cause of the ailment, which may be spasms of the coronary arteries. This new insight into the fundamental cause of heart disease could have profound ramifications for all of us.

In 1978, Italian doctors at the University of Pisa studied a group of high-risk candidates for heart attacks who had suffered symptoms of angina — chest pains caused by poor blood circulation. Doctors found that those patients who eventually suffered attacks had for some time previously been experiencing spasms of the coronary arteries — and that only later did blood clots form at the site of the spasms. At least for high-risk patients this evidence strongly suggests that spasms rather than blood clots are the primary cause of heart attacks.

If this theory is confirmed over the next few years by other researchers, it could indicate that doctors may have more success in lowering the risk of heart attacks by administering not anticoagulant drugs but drugs that ease coronary-artery spasms, and thus prevent blood clots from forming. Doctors at Harvard Medical School who have studied the new evidence from Italy claim that it could form the basis of a fresh approach to heart-disease treatment for the 1980s.

Alcohol

Evidence is accumulating that liquor — but no more than three "drinks" a day — may significantly decrease the risk of a heart attack. And California researchers have actually gone so far as to suggest seriously that "abstinence from alcohol may be a new risk factor" in developing heart disease.

California scientists at the Kaiser-Permanente Medical Center in Oakland recently studied the medical histories of 120,000 hospitalized patients. After allowing for such risk factors as age, obesity, hypertension, cigarette smoking, and blood-cholesterol levels, they concluded that moderate drinkers reported 30 percent fewer heart attacks than teetotalers. In a related study of 84,000 men and women, the scientists found that moderate drinkers also had slightly lower blood pressure, but total abstainers and heavy drinkers recorded higher blood pressure. Since then at least two studies have resulted in similar conclusions. According to a recently published study in the *New England Journal of Medicine*, Hawaiian researchers found that moderate drinkers shared a lower risk of heart attacks than heavy drinkers, but that drinkers-turned-teetotalers were the highest risks of all.

Why may alcohol decrease the risk of a heart attack? According to scientists, there are many possible reasons, from the most obvious — that a drink can relax you after a stressful day's work — to complex physiological factors that researchers are just beginning to comprehend. For instance, there is mounting evidence that alcohol in your blood may increase your body's production of the "good" high-density lipoproteins (HDL) that carry cholesterol to your metabolic furnace to be burned rather than allowing cholesterol to build up on artery walls.

While scientists pursue this interesting lead, you may choose to imbibe (if you already don't) a little beer, wine, or whiskey daily. Since the alcohol content of these beverages varies, nutritionist Dr. William J. Darby of Vanderbilt University in Nashville, Tennessee, defines a "drink" as a 1-ounce jigger of 80 proof spirits, a 3.5-ounce glass of wine, a 12-ounce mug of light European beer, or a 10-ounce mug of American beer.

Your Doctor's New Hypertension Drug

Though an occasional drink may lower your blood pressure slightly, a drug so new that it's still referred to by its research number, SQ 14225, may constitute the greatest breakthrough in curing hypertension — high blood pressure — in the last twenty years. It has none of the unpleasant side effects of the medicine currently prescribed for the common ailment of hypertension, which affects twenty-five million Americans, or 17 percent of all adults.

The drug is synthetically derived from a protein and is chemically similar to ingredients in snake venom that have proved effective in lowering high blood pressure. Drugs on the market work indirectly to reduce blood pressure, but SQ 14225 inactivates the hormone that causes blood vessels to constrict and stimulates production of the hormone that dilates vessels. It's this double action that endows the drug with its power and potential.

Researchers at Boston City Hospital have tested SQ 14225 on men and women with dangerously high blood pressure, some of whom had not responded to conventional drugs. In every case SQ 14225 reduced their blood pressure to the normal range. FDA tests are expected to confirm the benefits and safety of the drug, which could be approved and prescribed by doctors as early as 1983.

Your Body's Own Hypertension Drug

By the time SQ 14225 is commercially available doctors should be well into research on renin, a natural body chemical recently isolated in the laboratory. Researchers believe it may provide a prototype for a whole new class of drugs that would be safer and more effective in combating hypertension.

In 1978, two teams of researchers working separately extracted the chemical renin, an enzyme, from human kidneys. Our bodies produce renin in small quantities, and once it enters the blood stream it is converted to another chemical that constricts blood vessels and thus raises blood pressure. It is not entirely clear why certain people produce abnormally high amounts of renin, but stress, diet, and heredity are suspected as key factors. Dr. Eve Elizabeth Slater of Massachusetts General Hospital, one of the scientists who isolated renin, claims that the first practical spin-off of her discovery should appear around 1981 in the form of a simple, inexpensive blood test that for the first time will directly measure the amount of renin in the blood. This test will offer doctors a new method of evaluating a patient's risk of heart attack or stroke. Beyond that, doctors foresee a test to evaluate a child's renin-production mechanism to determine if he or she is a candidate for hypertension later in life. Alerted by such a warning, doctors would be able to take steps to reduce significantly the number of people who suffer debilitating paralysis or death caused by hypertension.

The Hard Work–Healthy Heart Link

No one is any longer surprised by the observation that people involved in more physically strenuous work suffer fewer heart attacks than more sedentary individuals. But the studies that have demonstrated this fact have yet to prove why hard work is beneficial for the heart. Some scientists, however, claim they have the first clues to the answer.

The connection between hard work and a strong heart has been suspected for decades and in recent years has been supported by at least six major studies. (The American Heart Association, though, points out that it is still unclear whether hard work itself benefits the heart, or if hard-working people generally have the kind of healthy dietary habits and life styles that make them less susceptible to heart attacks.) In one twenty-two-year-long study, scientists at the University of California at Berkeley examined the private lives and work habits of more than 3600 longshoremen between the ages of thirty-five and fifty-four. They found that those men employed for the most strenuous jobs had half as much risk of experiencing a fatal heart attack as did those who handled lighter work and had desk jobs, and who spent their leisure time watching television or fishing. The less active men, as well as the younger men who had not been working long at physically demanding labor, also were three times more likely to die suddenly and unexpectedly within an hour after the onset of an attack.

More recently, scientists from Harvard and two other universities concluded that men living at high altitudes in the mountains in New Mexico were less likely to die from heart attacks then men who resided closer to sea level. After taking into account such risk factors as smoking, obesity, and diet, they concluded that the thinner air at higher altitudes caused men both to work and to play more strenuously.

Cholesterol Carrier

There are probably several reasons why hard work keeps the heart, which after all is a muscle, young and strong. Doctors have known for years that people living at high altitudes are less likely to develop high blood pressure, and that when a person with high blood pressure moves to a higher altitude and acclimates to it, his or her pressure drops. But Dr. G. Harley Hartun of the Cardiac Rehabilitation Department at Methodist Hospital in Houston may be on to the most crucial link between hard work and a healthy heart.

Dr. Hartung studied a group of professional men and business executives. Some of his subjects jogged many miles a week, others ran infrequently, and some played golf and other sports that were not exertive enough to cause them to work up a sweat. Dr. Hartung found that the more active the man, the more his body produced the high-density lipoprotein that is believed to render cholesterol harmless. Even though the less active men tended to eat more high-fat foods and red meat, physical activity, not diet, was responsible for this increase in HDL. In their report to the American Heart Association, Dr. Hartung and his colleagues concluded that "the differences in HDL found are assumed to be directly related to physical activity habits of the groups." Thus, for the first time doctors have a glimpse into the complex biochemistry involved in the relation between strenuous, regular exercise and the lowered risk of heart disease.

Biofeedback for Your Heart

The same biofeedback techniques that have proved helpful to victims of migraines and ulcers, and that have even aided some cerebral palsy patients to regain use of their muscles, may also become a preferred treatment for atherosclerosis. In early tests, biofeedback is proving to be a highly effective method for increasing blood flow and thus diminishing the risk of heart trouble.

At Columbia University's College of Physicians and Surgeons, Dr. Kenneth Greenspan has originated an unorthodox program to combat heart disease. Three times a week for three months, he teaches victims of severe atherosclerosis to learn to relieve bodily stress through biofeedback techniques. First, they are taught how to relax their muscles, starting from the feet and progressing to the head. Next, using feedback sensors, they learn to direct blood flow to one hand. "This gives the person the confidence that he can master his own body," says Dr. Greenspan, "even functions he never thought he could control."

Dr. Greenspan is a firm believer that the daily stress of modern life is the single largest factor contributing to hardening of the arteris. "In the jungle, animals confronted with a stressful situation either fight or flee. We still have that primitive fight-flee cycle in us, but today there is little chance to resolve it. Consequently, most of us live in a continual state of chronic stress, which takes its toll on our cardiovascular system."

In 1978, in the first study of its kind, twelve men and women with severe atherosclerosis volunteered for Dr. Greenspan's biofeedback program. One fifty-five-year-old woman's arteries were so hardened that blood flow to her legs had been cut by 70 percent, and having to walk a few blocks caused her intense pain. Without drugs or surgery — "only teaching her how to relieve stress," says Dr. Greenspan — the woman increased her bloodflow by 40 percent and was able to begin jogging. In fact, all twelve patients in the program improved so dramatically that Physicians and Surgeons has begun a large-scale biofeedback study.

Dr. Greenspan hopes eventually to open a clinic in one wing of the hospital where people can, in effect, dilate their arteries by learning how to relax, then practice these techniques at home for twenty minutes a day. It's possible that by the mid-to-late 1980s many people seriously threatened by hardened arteries may be spared the additional dangers of surgery or drugs. Instead, they will be able to cure themselves with a remedy that is bound to include other beneficial effects on their life and longevity.

5

Dental Breakthroughs:
Saving Your Teeth

A Vaccine Against Tooth Decay

If your teeth already bear the gold and silver battle scars of tooth decay, you will not benefit fully from this breakthrough. But fillings may never mar the whites of your childrens' teeth. In ten years — fifteen at most — dentists believe they will be able to vaccinate infants against tooth decay just before they cut their baby teeth.

Tooth decay, or caries, is a disease of epidemic proportions. The U.S. Public Health Service estimates that every year America's 110,000 dentists fill half a million cavities, and that probably a billion teeth go untreated. Caries is caused almost entirely by a diet rich in refined sugars. Yet it's not the sugar itself that damages your teeth. Sugar, particularly sucrose, prepares a favorable environment for the bacterium *Streptococcus mutans* to flourish and colonize. The bacteria, collectively known as dental plaque, excrete two substances: a corrosive acid that dissolves tooth enamel, and a fiercely adhesive substance called dextran that permits the bacteria to stick to a tooth's bare surface while they bore their way in. Since caries is caused by a bacterium, scientists are optimistic about developing a vaccine against tooth decay.

Monkeys are already benefiting from one vaccine. They make excellent research subjects because they have the same number of teeth as we do, they develop caries in humanlike fashion, and they have a definite sweet tooth. In the early 1970s, Dr. William

Bowen of the Royal College of Surgeons in London inoculated monkeys with live strep cells, then fed them cookies, chocolates, and hard candies. Not only did the vaccinated monkeys develop fewer cavities after the first year, but five years later the vaccination was still protecting their teeth. More recently scientists at Guy's Hospital in London and the State University of New York in Buffalo have been testing a vaccine composed of dead strep cells. Monkeys given a single vaccination and then fed more typical human diets rich in canned, processed, and artificially flavored foods — all of which contain substantial amounts of refined sugar — have developed 60 to 85 percent less caries than monkeys not inoculated. Tests reveal that the vaccine does not produce antibodies that kill the *Streptococcus mutans;* rather, the antibodies prevent the groups of bacteria from forming the gluey dextran that enables them to adhere to the teeth.

In another five years, the dead strep vaccine may be perfected. Dr. Thomas Lehner, professor of oral immunology at Guy's Hospital, suspects that the whole cells of strep bacteria present in the vaccine could weaken human heart tissue. He is presently working with an extract from the bacteria that fights tooth decay and evidently has no influence on the heart. If animal tests scheduled for the early 1980s run smoothly, Lehner predicts the new vaccine could be tested on patients as early as 1985. By that time Dr. Bowen, who is now working for the National Institute of Dental Research in Bethesda, Maryland, hopes to have perfected a mouth wash that if used daily would be as successful against tooth decay as a vaccine.

Adults will be used as the first guinea pigs for both the vaccine and the mouth wash, and researchers expect to record the same wide degree of success found in monkeys. If the vaccine proves as effective as scientists believe it will be, by the end of the decade we may establish an immunization program in which infants are vaccinated against diphtheria, tetanus, whopping cough, and tooth decay at the same time.

Sweets That Don't Damage

While you're waiting for a vaccine against tooth decay, your teeth may be saved by a related breakthrough in the near future. At Michigan State University's College of Osteopathic Medicine, Dr. Jon Kabara is experimenting with the chemical Lauricidin. When eaten with sucrose-rich foods, Lauricidin neutralizes the effects of sugar on tooth decay. A nontoxic, germ-killing agent, Lauricidin is tasteless and has already been approved by the FDA as an additive in certain foods. Kabara says he still has to determine how much of the substance would have to be added to foods to counteract the effects of sugar, and how Lauricidin, a fatty compound, could affect the caloric content of foods. Since the FDA has already determined that Lauricidin is safe even when fed in large quantities to animals, it could show up in your canned fruits, pastries, and cereals in just a few years.

Health specialists are concerned that Lauricidin, as well as a vaccine or mouth wash against tooth decay, will be greeted by many people as a license for the gluttonous consumption of sweets. Since tooth decay constitutes one of the less injurious results to the body of refined sugar, many people may therefore be trading tooth decay for far more serious ailments.

Drilless Dentistry

Although the incidence of tooth decay may be greatly diminished, no vaccine or food additive will be able to wipe it out completely — at least, not in our lifetime. We shall occasionally be bothered by cavities, some people being more susceptible than others, but we won't ever again have to fear the pain of the dentist's drill. Doctors at Tufts Dental School have already perfected a chemical that literally sprays away tooth decay.

This painless, drilless method requires no anesthesia for even the biggest cavities. A chemical called GK-101 is drawn into a hand-held needle and squirted into the cavity. Within minutes, the decayed portion of the tooth breaks up and flakes away. You rinse your mouth with a disinfectant and spit out the decayed material. GK-101 has been tested on people with all sizes of cavities and has worked perfectly in nearly every case. In fact, only twice have Tufts dentists had to supplement the spray method with a small amount of drilling. In a few cases of internal cavities, drilling has been necessary to expose the decayed area enough for the chemical to work. Besides being painless, another advantage of GK-101 over drilling is that it removes only decayed material, where a drill also destroys a portion of the healthy part of the tooth. According to the FDA, which is currently testing GK-101, the chemical could be available by 1984.

6

Treatment Breakthroughs:

Conquering Pain, Obesity, and Your Body's Other Worst Enemies

Suffer No More

One of the most active areas of medical research in the 1980s will be the study and control of pain, be it chronic migraines, severe burns, injuries due to accidents, or the intense pain of cancer. Chances are that you, or someone you know, will be helped in the decade ahead by breakthroughs in pain research.

The pain-control revolution began in the early 1970s. Dolorologists (pain specialists) at the Stanford University School of Medicine implanted electrodes in the brains of patients whose excruciating pain was not relieved by drugs. An electrode was threaded down the back of a patient's head and into his chest, where it was connected to a receiver the size of a silver dollar. Whenever the patient felt pain, he placed a small transmitter next to his receiver, producing an electric current that interfered with the pain signals along nerves to the brain. Today, small, more convenient electric generators called Transcutaneous Nerve Stimulators (TNS), which are attached to the surface of the skin, are used by hundreds of people needing relief from pain. But they're not a panacea. Relief with a TNS is very temporary, lasting a few hours for some people, only minutes for others; and unfortunately, there are people for whom, inexplicably, a TNS has no effect at all.

The first step in conquering pain is to understand why electrical stimulation does work at all, and here dolorologists have recently made a breakthrough. Dr. Huda Akil of Stanford, who pioneered the original pain-relief work, has discovered that electrical stimulation causes the body to produce more of the brain proteins enkephalins, which are the body's natural painkillers. Dr. Akil has measured high levels of enkephalins in the spinal fluid of patients immediately after they have used their electric stimulators. It now appears that enkephalins block nerves running down the spinal cord that are carrying pain signals to the brain. The fact that pain can result from deficiencies in brain chemicals like enkephalins has given dolorologists hope of developing an arsenal of new drugs. (See *The Perfect Painkiller*, p. 122.)

Pain may not be completely conquered in the 1980s; there are still too many outstanding questions to be answered. For instance, do some of us have pain-prone personalities? There is evidence to support this possibility. Is there such a thing as pain memory? Some dolorologists believe that if, at one time in your life, you suffer truly intense pain, that experience may produce permanent changes in the nerve network to your brain, creating a pain memory that, like any memory, can be triggered years later by a traumatic — or pleasant — experience. In fact, this may be one cause of chronic pain. While other dolorologists pursue these issues, Dr. Akil continues to examine how electrical stimulation increases the production of enkephalins. Her discovery already offers dolorologists one explanation as to why electrical stimulation isn't effective for everyone: perhaps some of us can't produce as many enkephalins as others.

Measuring Hurt

How often have you suffered pain and wished to convey to your doctor or family how very badly it hurts? "It hurts more than . . ." "It's the worst, most intense pain . . ." Neither comparatives nor superlatives can adequately convey your suffering, and besides, there's always the chance that the people around you, perhaps even your doctor, may suspect you're exaggerating. Pain bears the dubious distinction in all of medicine of being the only ailment that cannot be measured objectively.

At least, this summarizes traditional medical opinion. But Dr. C. Richard Chapman of the University of Washington Medical School in Seattle believes he's discovered a method for measuring pain. He has used electric shocks to produce tooth pain in volunteers and then analyzed their brainwaves. The size of the brainwaves corresponded closely with the amount of pain the volunteers claimed they felt. More work is necessary to refine

Chapman's technique and to determine if it applies to all kinds of pain, wherever it may occur in the body. If, in the end, a brain-wave trace proves an accurate measure of pain, Dr. Chapman's discovery will stand as one of the biggest breakthroughs in the science of dolorology. By measuring pain, doctors may be less prone to pass off a patient's complaints as merely a psychological ruse for attention, and be compelled to adopt a more compassionate attitude toward suffering. By the end of the 1980s, Dr. Chapman's research may lead to a pain scale, perhaps with the extremes of zero for no pain to 100 for pain so intense that it causes a person to black out.

Eat and Grow Thin

Imagine indulging in your favorite foods and not gaining an ounce. Maybe even losing weight. This is not the goal of obesity research being conducted at the University of Illinois, but it could become one of its spin-offs — and very soon.

If you're seriously overweight, your doctor most likely has prescribed diet and exercise. You may have tried both, with only minimal success, and, like many heavy people, simply given up. Well, help is on the way — in the form of the most perfect slenderizing treatment imaginable. Dr. Sarfer Niazi, an Illinois pharmacologist, has found a thinning compound, perfluorooctyl bromide, that coats your gastrointestinal tract, temporarily blocking the absorption of food. The darkest chocolates, richest creams and pastries pass through your body without depositing a single calorie. After performing this miracle, the chemical, too, is eliminated, unchanged and unabsorbed. The perfluorooctyl bromide molecule is too large to enter the stomach lining or intestines. The drug has been tailor-made for those sixty million seriously overweight Americans whose lives are threatened by obesity, but it will be difficult to keep the drug away from all those obsessed with slender figures.

In one study, Niazi allowed rats a liberal diet, weighing them and their food intake every day. Rats not fed the chemical responded with weight gains of 8 percent a week; those fed the coating substance before each meal registered a 1 percent *decline* in weight. Niazi figures this result is the equivalent of a person losing eight pounds a week, regardless of his or her diet. The rats showed no adverse effects to the drug, and the wastes they excreted were normal, if rich in nutrients. Tests with rabbits and guinea pigs are running smoothly. Next, Niazi will try the slenderizing drug on chimpanzees. If it works, he'll schedule tests for people who are dangerously overweight.

The drug is expensive — about $50 a quart. But mass production could reduce the cost to a few pennies a dose. Niazi says that a dieter would have to take about 1.5 ounces before each meal. He emphasizes that the coating chemical should be used in tandem with a supervised regimen of diet and exercise, and that the slenderizer should not be viewed as a green light for indulging in food orgies. The Food and Drug Administration intends to double-check Niazi's findings to ensure that the drug does not enter the blood stream or accumulate in body tissues. If all goes well, perfluorooctyl bromide could be on the market — under a more appetizing name — by 1982. However, if Niazi has his way, you'll have to enter a hospital to get the drug. Otherwise, he feels, the temptation to gulp a few spoonfuls before every meal could be too great to resist. Unwittingly, people might diet themselves to death.

Spray Bandage

In the 1980s you'll be able to spray on a clear, thin bandage that has magic properties: it permits air and medications to pass through, while protecting against bacteria. It will be a convenience for many of us, but for those who suffer burns over much of their bodies, the spray bandage is a breakthrough that's truly a blessing.

A major burn is the maximum trauma that the human body can suffer and survive. To prevent infection, severe burns are now dressed with pigskin. It's effective, but the dressing must be changed two or three times a day. Also, pigskin bandage must be removed if medication has to be applied to the injured area, or if a doctor needs to check on the progress of recovery — all intensely painful procedures for a patient.

The new dressing — called a Hydron Burn Bandage — is the culmination of two decades of research and has already been tested at the Burns Institute of Shriners Hospital in Cincinnati, to the mutual satisfaction of doctors and patients. The bandage is formed by spraying a clear chemical solution over a wound, then sprinkling the area with a fine powdered polymer. The result is a biomaterial that "breathes" and stretches with the skin; it's invisible and porous, with the consistency of a soft contact lens. (Individual Hydron bandages have protected several burn patients for as long as twenty-seven days.) Since it is transparent, doctors can visually monitor healing, and the porous matrix of the bandage allows antibiotics to flow through. A good soaking in water and the Hydron bandage painlessly lifts off.

The Hydron Burn Bandage is undergoing tests at various burn centers around the country. Once it's approved by the FDA, the dressing could be sold in a spray can with an accompanying can of polymer powder. During the early 1980s it will be used exclusively in hospitals and burn centers, but before the end of the decade it could be stocked on drugstore shelves. You will be able to bandage, without pain, any burn, cut, or bruise that requires a few days of sterile environment.

Recapture Youth's Fitness

When young and in your healthy prime you'll bank some of your body cells as an investment in your future. Bottles of your white blood cells will be frozen, to be thawed decades later and injected into your body to fight infections and to ward off the diseases of old age. Periodic shots of your cells may even delay old age itself. It sounds like science fiction, but this youth bank of tomorrow could be made possible from advances in the 1980s in the burgeoning field of cryobiology.

Cryobiology is the tricky science of freezing cells. Tricky because if a cell is frozen too fast, ice crystals form inside and puncture the cell's walls. If a cell is frozen too slowly, salts build up and destroy it. The freezing process is further complicated by the fact that each different kind of cell in your body has its own optimum rate of freezing and thawing. However, several breakthroughs in cryobiology have already occurred. Today, red blood cells are routinely frozen at temperatures between −80° to −196° centigrade, and 200,000 units of frozen red cells are thawed each year for transfusions in the United States. Since sperm cells were first frozen in 1964, more than 3500 babies have been born from thawed sperm — some from sperm frozen for ten years. Because freezing and thawing sperm provide doctors with the time to check for genetic abnormalities or contagious diseases, frozen sperm have actually proved to be safer for conception than sperm direct from the testes. In 1979 a study at the University of Arkansas of more than 1000 children conceived from thawed sperm showed that fewer than 1 percent of them suffered birth defects, compared to 6 percent in the general population, and there were 6 percent fewer miscarriages among mothers impregnated with thawed sperm. But the biggest breakthroughs in cryobiology are yet to come.

Your White Cell Savings Account

In a few years cryobiologists at the Oak Ridge National Laboratory predict they'll be able to freeze your more fragile white blood cells, which are the soldiers that fight disease. This technique should promote a host of new medical treatments. By 1985, freezing white blood cells could be a lifesaving technique for leukemia victims. The Oak Ridge scientists claim that a leukemia patient whose disease is in remission could gradually build a reserve of frozen healthy cells that he could donate to himself if his condition worsened. A child with a genetically high risk of developing leukemia could start a healthy cell savings account that would support him in later life if he developed the disease.

All of us stand to benefit from frozen white blood cells. The scientists speculate that white and red blood cells donated and frozen when you're in your teens, and periodically injected into your body after you reach forty, could bolster your immune system, which naturally deteriorates with age. The red blood cells may improve the oxygen-carrying potential of your blood, increasing your stamina and lessening fatigue to such an extent that you would get a second wind in your sixties. Your young white blood cells might teach your older cells tricks they'd forgotten for fighting colds and other infections.

No respectable cryobiologist claims that weekly or monthly shots of young blood cells will turn your bald head hairy or smooth out laugh lines and crow's-feet. Such treatments could, though, significantly strengthen your defenses against such degenerative diseases of old age as diabetes, renal failure and kidney stones, arthritis, cancer (at least those kinds that may be caused by viruses or environmental antagonists), and certain heart problems. If transfusions of youthful cells really perform as cryobiologists anticipate, they will have effectively slowed down the aging process itself.

Organ Banks

Discoveries in cryobiology at a cellular level are paving the way for the breakthrough of the 1900s — organ banks.

Organs such as the liver, kidneys, or pancreas are hard to freeze because they contain a mixture of nerve, tissue, and blood vessel cells. Currently, most organs have to be transplanted within minutes or hours after they are removed from a deceased donor. As a consequence, doctors and recipients are often in the terrible position of waiting eagerly for an accident that will yield the necessary organ, and sometimes the organ arrives too late to do any good. Within our lifetime, however, these problems will be overcome, thanks to frozen-organ banks.

The first breakthrough is expected to occur with the freezing of kidneys. Researchers around the country are already transplanting thawed kidneys with increasing, though limited, success, and they have stumbled onto a new clue that may contribute to an important breakthrough. At Georgetown University, Dr. David Robinson has learned that freezing cells packed closely together, as they are in solid organs, sets off a destructive chain reaction: cells damaged by freezing release enzymes that destroy their healthy neighbors.

Scientists are now experimenting with different chemicals to protect individual cells while an organ is frozen. Oak Ridge cryobiologist Dr. Peter Mazur has found that the preservative dimethylsulfoxide works wonders on the pancreas. He has frozen the pancreases from rat fetuses, then thawed and transplanted them into adult rats. Not only did the pancreases function properly and produce insulin, but rats that had been experimentally turned into diabetics were, with the new pancreases, cured of the disease. Dr. Mazur asserts that one day transplanted pancreases may be used to cure human diabetics. Once they have mastered the technique of freezing kidneys and pancreases in the 1980s, cryobiologists predict the next breakthrough, perhaps to occur as early as the mid 1990s, will be the successful thawing of a frozen human heart. By the end of the century, banks of frozen organs will provide doctors the time they need to match the tissues of a donor and recipient in order to maximize the chances of a successful transplant.

Suspended Animation

Freezing body parts suggests an even more fantastic possibility. If a person develops an incurable disease, the entire body may be frozen in suspended animation and thawed — even decades later — when medical science is able to cure the ailment. Cryobiologists admit that this will not become a reality for many decades, for the technology required to freeze and thaw safely an organ as heterogeneous as the human body is staggering: every different body cell requires special treatment. By the time cryo-biologists acquire the medical know-how, there may be a pill to retard aging (see *Aging as a Curable Disease*, p. 135) and special diets to slow the deteriorative diseases of old age. And medical science may be so advanced, it will be able to cure most of the ailments plaguing us today. Those companies now freezing bodies immediately after death, promising restoration at a future date, are not credible. "Their freezing techniques have done extensive and irreparable cellular damage," warns one cryobiologist. "Resurrection, in the biblical sense of the word, would be easier than trying to repair billions and billions of destroyed cells."

Bloodletting's Back

You might think clearer, benefit from a sharper, more reliable memory — and the danger of a stroke or heart attack could be less — if your blood were thinner. If you're one of the many people who have unusually thick blood, within a decade your blood could be thinned by a modern version of the ancient practice of bloodletting.

Hemoglobin, the substance that supplies the blood with its hearty red color, also accounts for its thickness — and the thicker the blood, the more strain on your heart to pump it, and the less efficiently it delivers oxygen and nutrients throughout your body. At the Institute of Neurology in London, researchers discovered that bloodletting thins thick blood for a very simple reason: when the body loses blood, it acts immediately to replace the lost volume by appropriating water from body cells, thus diluting the blood. That's why blood donors often get thirsty. It takes a good while for the blood to replace red blood cells and thicken, so for a period of time after a person has lost blood, the remaining blood flows more freely through the body.

The London doctors, of course, did not *use* leeches in their experiments. They intravenously took a half-pint of blood at a time, over a period of a week, from people with unusually thick blood. The more blood patients lost, the lower their hemoglobin levels dropped, until eventually their blood had a normal viscosity; and the blood flow to the brain increased an average of 50 percent. The brain received not only more oxygen, but more of the nutrients that it converts into neurotransmitters, the chemicals that relay messages from neuron to neuron. Consequently, the patients may have experienced increases in mental ability, though the researchers were not testing for evidence of this.

Not all of us, of course, have abnormally thick blood. And the figures concerning the number of people who do are confusing. Several doctors are beginning to question whether today's accepted standard for blood viscosity and normal hemoglobin levels aren't a bit too high for modern-day living. To some doctors, the increase in stress-related heart attacks and strokes suggests that thinner blood might be more healthful, and lower standards may be necessary. If the American Medical Association lowers the norm for blood thickness, then thousands of us will automatically fall into the abnormally thick blood category. Such a shift is possible in your lifetime, and it could usher in bloodletting as a cure. If your doctor deems that the thickness of your blood jeopardizes your health, you may have to donate a few pints a year — solving your own problem while also increasing the stock in blood banks. Modern bloodletting remains in an experimental stage. But it may prove to be a very simple way to decrease your risk of a heart attack or stroke — and at the same time sharpen your mental acumen.

Your Hair Tells All

Your doctor routinely takes samples of your blood and urine as part of a complete physical examination, but he's missing a valuable diagnostic tool — your hair. By 1985, laboratories around the country may be analyzing strands of hair for evidence of diabetes and cystic fibrosis, as an aid in diagnosing schizophrenia, and, in a procedure that's sure to be controversial, for studying intelligence and learning disabilities in children.

Scientists' interest in hair originated with its use in solving crimes. Traces of chemicals in strands of hair found at the scene of a crime have since proved that hair can sometimes be as instructive as fingerprints in solving a murder. The techniques developed by forensic scientists have become so sophisticated that they are fostering a new area of diagnostic medicine. Many compounds, particularly trace elements, accumulate in hair at concentrations up to 100 times higher than in blood or urine, and some drugs show up in the hair shortly after they are swallowed and may remain there for months. In addition, hair is turning out to be an excellent barometer for measuring our exposure to environmental pollutants, and thus our risk for developing environmentally related diseases. The technical journal *Science* recently surveyed some of the breakthroughs in "hair diagnosis" on the horizon:

• Researchers at the Children's Hospital Medical Center in Boston have learned that children with cystic fibrosis have up to five times as much sodium in their hair as healthy children, and only about 10 percent as much calcium. Doctors hope to establish a ratio between these two elements in hair to help diagnose children for early signs of cystic fibrosis. Perhaps their discovery will eventually lead to a chemical treatment for the disease.

• If you're healthy, a strand of your hair contains about four times as much sodium as potassium. The opposite ratio can spell trouble. At the Massachusetts Institute of Technology scientists have found that there is much less sodium than potassium in the hair of people with celiac disease, a deficiency disorder caused by poor absorption of food in the intestine that can lead to severe malnutrition. When a celiac patient is treated with drugs, the ratio of sodium to potassium in the hair automatically returns to normal. This suggests a new way for doctors to monitor the speed and effectiveness of recovery.

The MIT researchers have also discovered trace-element imbalance for two other diseases. Hair from victims of phenylketonuria, a potentially fatal genetic disorder that makes a child's body accumulate toxic wastes, is deficient in magnesium and calcium, and causes mental retardation; and hair from victims of the severe malnutritional disease kwashiorkor, which results in a protuberant belly and stunted growth, contains an abnormally high concentration of zinc.

• Severe dietary deficiencies in zinc have long been blamed for retardation of growth and sexual development, but even slight deficiencies can have damaging effects. Scientists at Wayne State University Medical School have demonstrated that children registering low zinc levels in their hair suffer distortions and impairments in their sense of taste. Zinc supplements added to these childrens' diets restored their taste perception and the normal zinc levels in their hair.

• Evidence of diabetes has been discovered in hair. Doctors at the U.S. Department of Agriculture in Maryland have shown that the hair of children who develop diabetes is abnormally low in chromium, but the hair of adults who develop the disease contains normal chromium levels. This observation supports the currently popular medical belief that childhood and adult diabetes have different causes. The USDA doctors believe that hair analysis may be an accurate procedure for screening children with a tendency toward diabetes.

• Hair analysis may also help doctors diagnose and treat schizophrenia. Scientists at the University of Aston in Birmingham, England, have found that the hair of schizophrenics contains low concentrations of cadmium and manganese and high concentrations of lead and iron. No one knows how this imbalance develops, but it supports doctors' claims that manganese chloride is an effective treatment for some schizophrenics.

• I.Q. and the ability to learn new information may also be imprinted in the hair, according to Dr. Adon Gordus of the University of Michigan. He has found that the hair of students with high scholastic grades contained slightly, yet significantly, more zinc and copper, and less iodine, lead, and cadmium, than the hair of students with low grades. Though Gordus' findings are controversial, several scientists have shown that zinc deficiencies are linked with learning disabilities in animals and children. And recently scientists at McGill University in Montreal claimed that they had, with 98 percent accuracy, distinguished a group of normal children from those with learning problems simply by analyzing concentrations of fourteen elements in samples of their hair. The children with learning problems recorded higher levels of lead, cadmium, and manganese, and lower levels of lithium and chromium. Most impressive was the discovery that after these children underwent two years of behavioral therapy and mineral-supplemented diets, their learning abilities improved and the balance of trace elements in their hair returned to near-normal levels.

Hair analysis is still in its experimental stages, but it promises to constitute an important diagnostic tool — a strong complement to blood and urine analysis. Researchers are learning that more and more drugs accumulate in trace amounts in hair and remain there for months. If this is also true of the steroid drugs taken by many athletes, the 1984 Olympics may be the first of many sports contests where strands of an athlete's hair determine his or her eligibility to compete. Physicians may then play Delilah to the athletes' Samson.

Pulse-Power Therapy

Most medical treatments are based on altering the body's chemistry with drugs. In the decades ahead doctors will treat a wide range of problems by altering the body's internal currents with external electric fields. Sprained muscles, fractured bones, swollen joints, and perhaps even cancer, will be treated with these new electrotherapies.

Electromagnetic medicine seems a natural adjunct to drug therapy, since our body is as much an electrical power plant as a chemical factory. If anything, modern science has proved that the electrical nature of the body is more fundamental than its chemical nature, because all chemical reactions involving molecules and atoms require electrical potential to power them.

The idea that currents can cure bodily ills is hardly original. In the eighteenth century, Friedrich Anton Mesmer, a Viennese physician, theorized that a hypnotist forged a trance by "magnetizing" his subject, and many of Mesmer's followers treated the sick with jolts of electric current. Out of this bag of dubious and dangerous therapies one — electroshock therapy for severe mental depression — has survived to this day. The "current" doctors realized that electricity offered an untapped source for healing, but it is only very recently that scientists have begun to utilize that potential. Several new discoveries portend the breakthroughs we can expect in the decades ahead.

• At Manhattan's Columbia Presbyterian Medical Center, Dr. Andrew Bassett has demonstrated that quick pulses of current accelerate the rate at which bone fractures mend. The current seems to boost the body's own healing process to forge firm, sturdy bones. Another New York physician, Dr. Abraham Ginnesburg, has found that the calcium that often builds up around a swollen joint when a person is suffering from bursitis can be broken down and eliminated from the body by the use of electric-current therapy, thus lessening the tenderness of the inflamed joint. Their experiments have encouraged a number of leading hospitals to use pulses of high-frequency electromagnetic fields for treating sprained ankles, strained shoulder muscles, and swollen joints.

• Bones are not the only parts of your body that respond favorably to electric fields. At Howard University in Washington, D.C., Dr. E. B. Chung has demonstrated that pulsed electromagnetic fields can reduce the swelling of tissues bruised in accidents or lacerated by surgery. He has also found that pulsed EM therapy, as the treatment is referred to, accelerates the growth of new skin over burned areas of patients' bodies. After a single EM treatment, burn patients experience tremendous relief from pain. It seems this relief is due to the reduction in excess fluids that accumulate in tissues traumatized by burns. Just how pulsed EM therapy accomplishes this feat is one of the mysteries Dr. Chung intends to solve in the next few years.

What is a pulsed electromagnetic field? And why must it be pulsed — broken — instead of continuous? The most popular EM treatment relies on a device called a Diapulse to generate high-frequency radio waves similar to those that carry television pictures. If the energy in the waves was delivered continuously to a portion of the body, a buildup of heat would burn the surrounding tissues. When the energy is transmitted to the injured area in rapid bursts of 80 to 600 pulses a second, the heating effect is avoided and treatment time can be greatly increased. With the Diapulse device the pulses emanate from a large circular disk placed next to your body, and the only sensation you may feel is a slight tingle.

To Speed Up Healing

Scientists experimenting with the new therapy are still faced with the problem of explaining how pulsed electromagnetic fields produce their healing biological effects. Most of them feel that the answer lies in first understanding how electrons and charged particles called ions move in and out of the body's cells. Cells normally have an electric potential that is negative on the inside of the membrane wall and positive on the outside. Externally applied EM fields seem to alter the membrane potentials and force otherwise reluctant electrons and ions through cell walls, expediting healing. The most far-reaching theory of membrane potentials has been proposed by Dr. Clarence Cone of NASA's Langley Research Center, in Virginia. He believes that the lower the membrane potential of a cell, the more likely it is that the cell will divide and proliferate new healthy cells. If ongoing experiments prove Cone's elegant hypothesis to be correct, it would explain why nerve and muscle cells, which have high membrane potentials, are so reluctant to regenerate, and why malignant cells, which have very low membrane potentials, multiply and spread wildly. Cone is optimistic that electric fields could raise the membrane potential of cancerous cells, thus halting their spread. From work progressing in the opposite direction, there is already evidence that pulsed EM waves can stimulate certain kinds of nerve cells to regenerate, offering hope for some victims of paralysis and other neurological disorders.

Electromagnetic medicine is a nascent science, but even at this early stage there is every reason to believe that during the next two decades it will mature into a powerful medical tool, producing an abundance of new therapies that are extremely safe and very inexpensive to administer. (See *Ions for Your Health*, p. 161; and *Fields to Modify Your Behavior*, p. 165.)

Growing New Limbs

By applying gentle, steady, and very weak electric currents, doctors in just one decade may be able to help the body regrow damaged or diseased joints and bones, and straighten deformed spines. A few decades beyond lies the very real possibility for the regeneration of lost fingers and toes, entire arms and legs.

Any scientist who has watched a newt produce a missing arm or leg has wondered if the process could be duplicated in humans. If limb regeneration could be forced to occur in animals more evolved than the newt, then certainly it could be possible for us, too. With that belief as their lodestar, biologists in the mid 1970s achieved major breakthroughs in regeneration with animals. Using continuous electric currents, they succeeded in inducing frogs to grow back severed toes, then entire legs. Rat amputees regrew arms from the shoulder to the elbow — with cartilage, bone, nerves, and muscles in perfect anatomical precison. Biologists discovered that the healing currents always had to be *pulled out* of the stump in order to coax regrowth; inward-flowing current actually caused degeneration. So successful were these experiments that the research challenge for the 1980s is to understand why some animals spontaneously regrow limbs while others need external currents to accomplish regrowth. This will be the first step toward achieving the regeneration of lost human limbs.

Various clues are already emerging. Recently three biologists at Purdue University found that amphibians spontaneously grow new limbs through the use of electric currents that naturally travel along the surface of the animal's skin. These skin currents course along the limbs of newts, increasing fiftyfold along the stump of amputated limbs. As the limb begins to regenerate spontaneously, the skin currents gradually weaken, and by the time the limb has fully regrown the currents have returned to their normal values.

What is the source of these natural, miraculous currents?

Until a few years ago biologists thought these currents were generated by nerve cells and that they peaked when nerves were shocked by injury or amputation. Now they know that the newts' natural regeneration currents spring from concentrations of sodium in the skin covering a stump. By alternately increasing and decreasing sodium concentrations, biologists have measured a sort of yo-yo acceleration and deceleration of limb growth.

Human Currents

Might there be natural skin-driven currents in us? Maybe they are so weak that, even shocked by bodily injury or amputation, they cannot promote healing. Perhaps they can be strengthened with external electromagnetic fields or by an increase in the sodium content of a wound or stump.

Several researchers are making progress in these areas. Dr. Carl Brighton of the University of Pennsylvania School of Medicine has had excellent results from using electric currents to heal the broken bones of elderly patients. Brighton's method involves implanting several Teflon-coated electrodes into a fractured bone before the limb is set in a cast. Wires connect the electrodes to a power source, and for about twelve hours a day weak currents of 20 microamperes travel down the electrodes and "cement" the fracture together. Dr. Brighton believes the electricity activates certain bone cells called osteoblasts, which, in younger people, cause the accumulation of calcium and other minerals that act to cement broken bones. In treating more than 200 patients, Dr. Brighton has achieved a success rate of 84 percent.

Dr. Robert Becker, a pioneer in the field of cell regrowth biology and chief of orthopedic surgery at the Veterans' Administration Hospital in Syracuse, New York, has had even more success with electrotherapy. In patients whose fractured leg bones would not heal because they had diabetes, Dr. Becker has been able to prevent leg amputations by implanting electrodes into the fractures; after several applications of current the fractures healed and the legs were saved. From his experiments with animals he believes that electric currents may one day be used to regenerate damaged heart muscles, lessening the need for risky heart surgery and decreasing the incidence of heart attack. The regeneration of human limbs, claims Dr. Becker, will surely follow.

One encouraging observation about our potential to regenerate limbs to some degree came recently from British physicians. Two infants lost their fingers in an accident immediately after birth; as the babies grew, so did new fingers. At a very early age the human body apparently has the capacity for regrowth; what remains to be discovered is how to stimulate that possibility later in life when it may be needed.

While some researchers have begun to measure the levels of sodium in both healthy legs and stumps of amputees, Dr. Becker is concentrating his efforts on a problem that may be solved in the next few years: the regeneration of segments of a paralyzed patient's spinal cord. The spinal cord in humans does not regenerate at all. Once it is severed, the person is paralyzed for life. Experiments are just beginning, but Dr. Becker hopes to show by the mid 1980s that paraplegic dogs and monkeys can be returned to normal health through electrodes implanted in the spinal cord that electrically stimulate the repair and regrowth of nerves and vertebrae. If the experiments are successful and without adverse side effects, the technique could be attempted on humans by the end of the decade. It may be that human longevity will be advanced not through bionic research and artificial parts but with the aid of regenerated natural parts — bones, limbs, and even major internal organs.

Saving Your Brain

Strokes, heart attacks, or drownings assault the brain by depriving it of vital oxygen. When that happens the brain swells, pushing against the skull and increasing the risk of permanent brain damage or death. These incidents are usually fatal, because treatment must be swift, and attempts to reduce swelling with injections of steroid hormones or by surgical removal of portions of the skull often fail to save the brain from neurological damage. In a few years, however, rescue may be achieved by administering common barbiturates immediately after an accident or seizure.

The new breakthrough in using barbiturates to thwart swelling came from a simple medical observation: the brains of people who had committed suicide with larges doses of barbiturates didn't swell. This was the starting point for current experiments on people whose conditions appear hopeless. At one California hospital, anesthesiologist Dr. Harvey Shapiro and neurologist Dr. Lawrence Marshall gave forty-five comatose patients, who were being sustained on mechanical respirators, large intravenous doses of phenobarbital for up to two weeks. In all cases, X rays revealed that the swelling subsided. Twenty patients previously considered incurable recovered with no neurological injuries; six more revived with only moderate disabilities. Barbiturates administered to patients dying from brain injuries decreased the mortality rate at the hospital by a stunning 65 percent. In related work, Dr. Julian Hoff, a California neurosurgeon, has successfully used barbiturates on patients undergoing surgery to correct cerebral aneurysms, the weak bulging pouches in the walls of brain arteries that constitute the second major cause of strokes. Without the barbiturates, Dr. Hoff believes, many of his patients would have died.

Neurologists at several hospitals are experimenting with barbiturates in order to understand how they save the brain. Dr. Shapiro thinks they may help by constricting the brain's blood vessels, or by reducing the chemical activity of brain cells, thus lowering their need for oxygen. Several more years of research are necessary before barbiturate therapy can become standard practice, but by the end of the 1980s it could be a successful medical procedure for saving thousands of people from crippling impairments, retardation, and even death.

Aspirin to Prevent Strokes

From 1971 to 1977, Dr. Henry Barnett of the Neurological Sciences Clinic of the University of Western Ontario experimented with 585 stroke victims, two thirds of them men. After testing various medications, he finally concluded that four aspirins a day reduced by almost 50 percent the chance of a high-risk patient suffering a second stroke.

Dr. Barnett believes that aspirin prevents platelets in the blood from forming clots, which can lodge in a crucial artery and cause a stroke. Aspirin, however, did not reduce the risk of strokes in women, presumably because female sex hormones alter its action.

Dr. Barnett announced his discovery in February 1978, and it immediately touched off a rash of experiments to determine the true effectiveness of aspirin. The results of these studies are expected in the early 1980s. If they document the fact that aspirin does substantially reduce the risk of a second stroke, then researchers will attempt to answer an even more important question: Can a few aspirins a day prevent a first stroke?

Awakening the Dead

Defining the state of death can be an imprecise business. At present, one major criterion is an EEG (electroencephalograph) trace that records flat brainwaves for twenty-four hours. However, another device much more sensitive than the EEG can detect signs of life in people ordinarily considered dead by clinical standards. One doctor has already awakened the "dead," and in the decade ahead other physicians are sure to follow suit.

Brain damage, by contemporary definition, requires that a doctor declare a patient's brain irreversibly damaged by massive injury. It's not an easy determination to make, and many doctors refuse to give up hope that a patient may awaken even though his brain registers no activity.

At the College of Medicine of the University of California at Irvine, neurologist Dr. Arnold Starr has developed a sensitive audio device that measures signals from deep within the brain. Electrodes precisely like those used in an EEG are attached to a patient's scalp and ear lobe, then wired to a sophisticated audio-tracking system 1000 times more sensitive to the brain's currents than the standard EEG. A set of headphones over the patient's ears feeds a series of loud, rapid clicks, and a computer searches out the sound and tracks it through the brain to determine whether the brain is actually dead or merely idling at a rate too slow for the EEG to measure. "This is the first time," says Dr. Starr, "that we've been able to get feedback from the depth of the brain, and with a procedure that takes only about four minutes."

Dr. Starr has tested his device on patients who by EEG evidence were dead. "In several cases where the patient appeared to be brain dead, we detected auditory brain-stem response," he says. "On further examination we found that these patients had taken overdoses of drugs. They eventually awakened and recovered." In every case signals from deep within the brain do not mean that a comatose patient has the potential to wake up; that's for a neurologist to decide. But Starr's audio device may soon be coupled with the EEG to provide physicians with a more reliable standard of brain death.

The device also has other important applications. It can determine whether a person is unconscious as a result of poison, a blood clot, or a brain tumor; an EEG cannot make these distinctions. By 1985 the audio device may be used to test the hearing of newborn infants. The detection of a hearing weakness early in a baby's life can prevent learning problems later on, and avoid the tragic diagnosis that a child is mentally retarded when, in fact, the child is only hard of hearing.

7

Gene Breakthroughs:
How You'll Change Your Past and Shape Your Future

Gene Analysis to Wipe Out Disease

In a few years doctors — merely by examining single genes — ought to be able to test you or your unborn baby for hundreds of genetically caused diseases. By the end of the decade computers could rapidly perform these tests on a massive scale to provide highly detailed analyses of a fetus's genetic past and future. Several scientists have predicted that this technique could eliminate all genetic diseases by the end of the century. "The isolation of genes and the ability to manipulate them puts us at the threshold of a new form of medicine," says Dr. Paul Berg, a biochemist at Stanford University.

The National Institutes of Health estimate that thirteen million Americans currently suffer from diseases caused by defective genes, and that 6 percent of all babies born each year suffer from genetic problems. These range from such ailments as muscular dystrophy, cystic fibrosis, Huntington's disease, hemophilia, and Down's syndrome (commonly called mongolism), to inherited ethnic diseases like sickle-cell anemia in blacks, Cooley's anemia in Mediterraneans, striatonigral degeneration (a neurological disorder) in Portuguese, and Tay-Sachs in Jews. Genetic propensities for diabetes, epilepsy, high blood pressure, and certain kinds of mental illness are also inherited. Doctors have identified more than 2000 genetic diseases and estimate there may be many others yet to be discovered.

The drive to eliminate genetic diseases has already begun. Today there are over 200 genetic-counseling centers in the United States for (1) genetic analysis of adults who wish to become parents, (2) fetal analysis, and (3) immediate postnatal analysis of infants. At present, most gene analysis is based on blood samples — a procedure not entirely free of danger for the fetus. There is, however, a safer, relatively new, and virtually painless method of fetal analysis called amniocentesis. In this procedure, usually performed on a woman in her sixteenth week of pregnancy, a long needle is inserted into the amniotic cavity of the womb to withdraw a sample of the amniotic fluid. This fluid surrounds the developing fetus and contains cells shed by the baby, thus providing samples of the genes. A large clinical study by NIH scientists in 1978 concluded that amniocentesis is safe for both mother and child.

Cutting DNA

Once a gene sample is obtained, it must, of course, be analyzed. Though present laboratory techniques can identify only about 80 of the more than 2000 known genetic diseases, researchers could soon be identifying many more as the result of a recent breakthrough made by doctors from the Harvard and Yale medical schools and the Children's Hospital Medical Center in Boston. These doctors have developed the first clinical technique that permits examination of a single gene — a remarkable achievement, considering that in each body cell there are roughly 50,000 genes that determine a person's hereditary traits.

The new technique is possible through the use of what are called restriction enzymes, which allow doctors to clip a string of genes (a piece of DNA chain) into thousands of tiny fragments, and then radioactively label each fragment in order to examine individual genes for missing parts or flaws in the genetic code. The genes can be obtained from a blood test or, in the case of a fetus, from the amniotic fluid. The restriction enzymes have the magical property of being able invariably to cut a string of genes in precisely the same place, a feat that has earned them the title of the "chemical knives" of genetic research, and won for their discoverers — Dr. Werner Arber, of the University of Basel, and Drs. Daniel Nathans and Hamilton Smith, of Johns Hopkins University — the 1978 Nobel prize in medicine. At present, scientists have catalogued at least eighty restriction enzymes that sever DNA at various sections of its chain.

So far, the Boston scientists have used restriction enzymes to

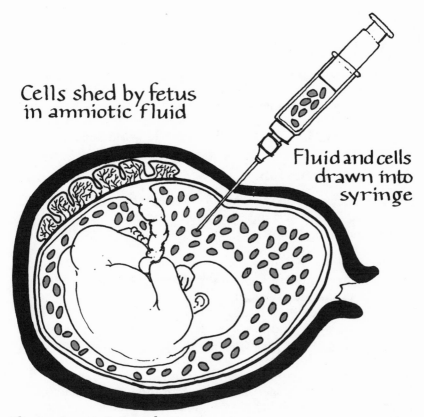

Cells shed by fetus in amniotic fluid

Fluid and cells drawn into syringe

The Amniocentesis Procedure

A hypodermic needle inserted into an expectant mother's uterus is used to withdraw cells shed into the amniotic fluid by the growing fetus. The cells are then tested for defects in chromosomes and genes. Amniocentesis is regarded as a safe procedure for both mother and child, and it currently can detect about eighty hereditary diseases.

diagnose clinically two common types of anemia, but they believe that by relying on various radioactive-labeling probes they eventually may be able to detect nearly all genetic defects. Their technique could make amniocentesis, which is now practiced in a few hospitals, an indispensable medical procedure within a few years. If a prenatal analysis uncovered severe gene abnormalities in a fetus, the mother could elect to have an abortion. And if a doctor failed adequately to advise a pregnant patient that her fetus contained seriously defective genes and she subsequently bore a child with birth defects, there is a chance that the doctor could be held liable for the special costs of a lifetime of care for the child.

The number of genetic-counseling centers in the United States is expected to more than double by 1985, and the Boston researchers consider their gene-visualizing technique especially promising for diagnoses in the developing countries, where hereditary diseases are more common than in the United States. In fact, they envision international analysis centers that could quickly analyze blood or amniotic fluid samples flown in from hospitals in the most remote corners of the world.

Genes and Your Job

Computerized gene analysis could one day inform you if you have "sensitized" genes and therefore should avoid certain jobs, living environments, or a marriage that would increase the risk of disease for you or your children.

At NASA's Jet Propulsion Laboratory in Pasadena, California, scientists are designing a computer that will be able to analyze a fetal blood sample, then print out a complete picture of the baby's genetic health or abnormality, as well as his or her susceptibility to various diseases in later life. On a smaller scale, Dr. Robert Ledley of the National Biomedical Research Foundation has already developed a prototype of a gene-analyzing computer. His experimental device can study a human chromosome (which contains thousands of genes) in less than thirty seconds and compare it against normal-chromosome charts that have been programed into the computer's data bank. Though Ledley's and the JPL's computers work with blood samples, they could be adapted to analyze genes from amniotic fluid. Once scientists identify the function of each gene — a task that will be facilitated by the discovery of additional restriction enzymes — a computer gene analysis could intimately acquaint a prospective mother with her unborn baby. A mother could find out her baby's eye and hair colors, skin tone, potential health strengths and weaknesses, and possibly even the genetic component of intelligence a full six months before giving birth.

Eventually, we may all benefit from computer gene analysis, for scientists are learning that some of us have greater propensities than others for certain occupation-related diseases.

Lung Disease

There is strong evidence, for instance, that an inherited deficiency of a body chemical called alpha-antitrypson predisposes people to a variety of lung ailments. Workers deficient in alpha-antitrypson who must be around certain chemicals suffer a high rate of emphysema. In California, hundreds of teen-agers recently found deficient in alpha-antitrypson have been warned of the increased hazard of cancer from smoking.

Sex Diseases

Researchers believe that genetic predisposition may explain why long-term exposure to low levels of anesthetic gases in operating rooms causes reproductive problems, including painful menstruation, infertility, and miscarriage, in some women nurses and doctors more than in others.

Cancer

British researchers have evidence that people carrying the inherited blood antigen B27 may be particularly sensitive to the carcinogenic effects of asbestos. The B27 antigen also appears to predispose a person strongly to the crippling disease of ankylosing spondylitis, which attacks the spinal cord. Dr. William Gough of the Cornell Medical Center of New York Hospital advises that children of parents with ankylosing spondylitis who have the B27 antigen should "avoid occupations such as driving, dentistry, surgery, and professional athletics, which are likely to place excessive strain on the back."

• • •

Computer gene analysis on a large scale raises preplexing moral questions. Will those of us with certain "defective" or "sensitized" genes be stigmatized by society? Discriminated against in jobs? Forbidden to marry? And what about the expectant mother who does not like the gene report on her fetus? If the report predicts that her baby has a high potential to develop lung cancer at age forty or that he or she carries the B27 antigen or won't have the desired coloring, should she be allowed to have an abortion? With computer gene analysis perhaps a decade away, these questions are of particular relevance. They will have to be resolved before the procedure becomes a routine practice in pregnancy.

Gene Therapy

"It is now conceivable that not within 100 years, not within twenty-five years, but perhaps within five to ten years, certain inborn errors of metabolism will be treated or cured by the administration of the particular gene that is lacking." That is the prediction of Dr. Theodore Friedmann of the University of California's School of Medicine in San Francisco. If gene analysis can't eliminate genetic diseases, Dr. Friedmann believes that gene therapy can — by employing new techniques that allow doctors to cut out "bad" genes and insert fresh genetic information in their place. Gene therapy promises to be one of the most powerful, beneficial techniques of genetic engineering.

Although gene therapy is in its infancy, genetic material from animals and man has been successfully transplanted into bacteria to produce true chimeras — organisms endowed with the genetic characteristics of two unrelated species. Through such techniques, bacteria have been formed to produce rat insulin, human brain hormone, and human insulin. A major advance in gene therapy occurred in 1978, when Dr. Paul Berg accomplished the first successful transplant of a functioning gene from one mammalian species to another, using recombinant DNA techniques. Through genetic transfer, Dr. Berg got the cells of an African green monkey to produce the blood hemoglobin of a rabbit. (Because the DNA code is universally democratic, governing paramecia as well as presidents, the transfer of genetic information between species is possible, and can illuminate the way in which genes store information.)

The Perfect Cure

The goal of recombinant DNA research, of course, is not to produce exotic chimeras; one of its eventual aims is to implant functioning, healthy human genes into genetically defective cells. Researchers suggest that the first clinical breakthrough in human gene therapy will occur with the implantation of insulin genes into the body cells of diabetics, enabling them to produce their own insulin without the necessity of daily shots. Other diseases that may be cured by gene therapy are hemophilia, Tay-Sachs, and PKU (phenylketonuria), which occurs in infants who lack an enzyme necessary to break down phenylalanine, an amino acid in many common foods.

Once one enzyme-deficiency disease is conquered by gene therapy, researchers believe it will be relatively easy to cure the more than fifty other such known ailments. There is optimism among biochemists that once they understand the genetic flaw that causes cancer, gene therapy could become the preferred cure. Scientists are now experimenting with ways in which healthy, new genes can best be inserted into body cells, where they would take command over errant genes. When that technique is perfected, gene transplants could be elevated to become the ultimate cure-all.

Any therapy so powerful, however, has its dangers. Weeding out "bad" genes would purify our human gene pool. Since part of the evolutionary strength of a species lies in the diversity within its genes, a pool too pure could weaken our resistance to environmental diseases. Dr Friedmann believes that the use of gene therapy to cure the more than four million diabetics in the United States "might appreciably affect the overall quality of the gene pool." Thus, instead of tailoring a race of "perfect" people, we could produce beautiful offspring prone to illness. Most likely, government controls on gene therapy will be initiated in the early 1980s. Perhaps a decade later gene therapy would be a fairly common procedure in treating many genetic diseases. Though blood transfers and organ transplants are responsible for saving many lives today, gene therapy may become the preferred and far more effective lifesaving technique in the very near future.

Drugs from Genes

Within a few years biologists, instead of chemists, will be producing our new miracle drugs, and genetic-engineering techniques will make it possible to mass produce and, consequently, sell at inexpensive rates drugs that to date are rare and costly.

By cleverly plugging human genes into bacteria, scientists have already coerced bacteria to produce human insulin and the brain hormone somatostatin. That's particularly encouraging for diabetics whose lives depend on daily doses of insulin extracted from cattle and pig pancreases. The extraction process is expensive, and as the number of diabetics increases, doctors fear the supply of animal insulin will drastically dwindle. What's more, animal insulin is only 98 percent pure and sometimes causes allergic reactions; on the other hand, bacteria-produced human insulin is 100 percent pure and should be tolerated to a greater degree.

Scientists are continually experimenting with different techniques to coax bacteria to produce drugs. Some researchers start directly with human genes, but the California scientists who produced somatostatin and insulin started by creating synthetic genes. They synthesized the fragments of human DNA that are known to manufacture insulin, then inserted the fragments into bacteria that in turn produce insulin.

All of the techniques involve the delicate splicing of human genetic information into the DNA chain of a simple bacterium — almost always *Escherichia coli,* which is located in the human intestine. The bacteria are then programed to manufacture millions of molecules of hormones and drugs. In 1979 scientists at the University of California School of Medicine in San Francisco developed bacteria capable of producing human pituitary growth hormone, which is used in age-retardation research and for the treatment of growth deficiencies in children. This breakthrough offers particular promise, since the hormone — currently extracted from the pituitaries of people who recently died — has always been in very short supply. Next, researchers hope to engineer bacteria to provide clotting factor for hemophiliacs, and eventually new vaccines, vitamins, and antibiotics, all tailor-made for the human body by information already stored in our genes.

When will you be able to buy bacteria-produced drugs?

At the genetic-engineering firm of Genentech, Inc., the researchers responsible for the breakthroughs in brain hormone and insulin are gearing up for the mass production of insulin. By their most optimistic estimate, they could have huge vats of bacteria churning out insulin by 1982. But prior to marketing the product, they must perform animal tests with the insulin, and follow up with clinical safety studies on people. The first bacteria-produced human insulin may be commercially available by the end of the decade; the human growth hormone shortly afterward. Other bacteria-produced drugs should begin appearing in the mid 1990s.

New Life Forms

In addition to producing new drugs, bacteria are being designed to perform a variety of tasks. Dr. Ananda Chakrabarty, a microbiologist at General Electric, has already created a strain of bacteria that gobbles up industrial oil spills, and scientists at the Upjohn Company have engineered a strain, also nonexistent in nature, that produces high yields of the antibiotic lincomycin. Before the decade is over, scientists hope to produce special nitrogen-fixing bacteria that would live in the roots of crops, virtually eliminating the need for fertilizer.

The legal battle lines are now being drawn, and important issues are at stake. May a biologist patent a new organism? Who should set guidelines for creating new life forms? Who should determine the new kinds of life that are to be created? Even before these basic issues are resolved, Eli Lilly, Abbott Laboratories, Hoffmann-LaRoche, and other drug companies are spending millions of dollars to originate the new life forms that promise to revolutionize the chemical and pharmaceutical industries. Sizing up the moneymaking potential of these life forms, *Fortune* magazine predicts the field will yield a "multi-billion dollar industry," and *Business Week* says: "The ultimate impact on the chemical and pharmaceutical industries could be similar to that which followed when an understanding of solid state physics was brought to electronics: Genetic engineering is, in effect, ready to graduate from the vacuum tube to the transistor."

Exotic Hybrids

A green bean with the protein content of a steak. A noncholesterol breakfast cereal with the nutritional value of eggs made by crossbreeding a chicken with a barley plant.

By the use of the latest techniques of genetic engineering, exotic plant-plant, animal-plant — and even people-plant — chimeras are already being produced in laboratories. According to a government study, agricultural technology has "exhausted the previously existing backlog of basic research," and the hope for feeding the world's future populations lies in the genetic engineering of plants. The most immediate goals of the new genetic agriculture are to develop crops that manufacture their own fertilizer, and plants that are resistant to weed-killers and specific diseases. Next comes the quest for ingenious plant-plant hybrids that combine the nutritional value of two or more plants in one crop; then, animal-plant hybrids genetically tailored to the nutritional needs and metabolism of animals and man.

Cell "fusionists" have already cleared several of nature's biggest hurdles. By combining genetic material from different cells, within the last few years they have crossed protein-rich soybeans with carbohydrate-rich corn, barley, peas, and carrots, in an attempt to pack a full, balanced meal into a single crop. No one has yet tasted this genetic succotash, because scientists have succeeded only in growing the cells in formless clumps, not full plants. But full plants, claim plant biologists, are no more than five years in the future. A breakthrough that may occur even sooner is the profitable marriage between soybean and wheat plants. Soybeans extract directly from the atmosphere some of the nitrogen plants need to grow, and wheat plants need ni-

trogen-rich fertilizer; so a soybean-wheat hybrid would be a nutritional bonanza and could save millions of dollars a year now
spent on fertilizers. Summing up the goals of genetic agriculture,
Michigan State University plant scientist Dr. Peter Carlson says,
"This is a long-range technology, and the big payoffs may not
occur for a decade or more. But by attempting to turn biology
into a technology, we are creating more genetic variability, and
the name of the game is genetic variability if we are to meet the
food problems of the decades ahead."

People-Plant Hybrids

Although the very idea conjures up horrific images, scientists are
already making progress in creating plant-mammal hybrids.
Hungarian scientists have fused human cells with those of carrots, and researchers at the University of London have mated the
red blood cells from hens with yeast cells. At the Brookhaven National Laboratory in Upton, Long Island, Dr. Harold Smith has
fused human cells with those of a tobacco plant. The Brookhaven
report on the experiment states, "The fusion process was fairly
simple, just a matter of mixing the two cell preparations together
and incubating them at room temperature with polyethylene gly-
col (PEG)." PEG acts like a glue, and once the walls of two cells
have been chemically stripped away, PEG fuses the genetic material of the two cells into a single body. "These 'tobacco-man fusion cells' not only survive in the liquid growth medium," the
Brookhaven report continues, "but grow back the plant cells'
walls. However, careful analysis clearly reveals that the human
nucleus remains." Such hybrid cells divide, and biologists think
it's only a matter of time before they'll be able to coax these
chimeras to grow into beneficial plants.

What can we gain from the union between human cells and
plant cells?

No one expects these hybrids to grow hands or feet. In fact, all
the human DNA does not survive multiple cell divisions, so the
hybrid is actually more plant than man (or woman, in the Brookhaven case). At the moment scientists hope to experiment with
such hybrids to isolate and study the behavior of single human
genes. In the long run, they anticipate that people-plant hybrids
will retain sufficient amounts of human DNA to produce human-
type enzymes and drugs. Just as bacteria have been persuaded to
produce valuable human insulin and hormones, scientists expect
that in the future certain human hormones and enzymes will be

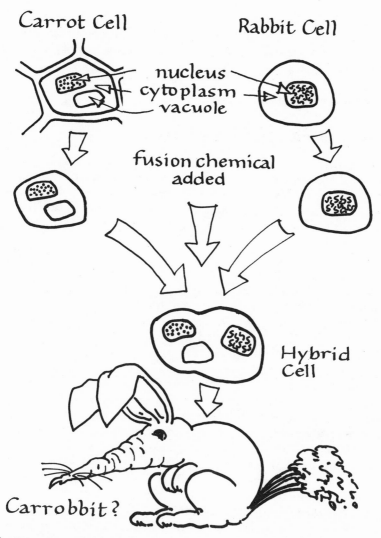

Carrot Cell **Rabbit Cell**

nucleus
cytoplasm
vacuole

fusion chemical added

Hybrid Cell

Carrobbit?

The New Cross-Breeding

Exotic plant-plant, animal-plant, and people-plant hybrids have already been made in laboratories. Cells of protein-rich soybeans have been crossed with cells of carbohydrate-rich corn in an attempt to pack a balanced meal into a single crop. Red blood cells from chickens have been crossed with yeast cells, and human cells have been fused with cells from carrots and tobacco plants. To date, such hybrids have grown into formless clumps, preserving the genetic contributions of both primary cells. The goal of cell-fusion biology is to produce crops with extraordinary nutritional value, as well as plants that can be harvested for the human enzymes, hormones, and vitamins they produce.

nurtured in greenhouses and harvested from hybrid plants' leaves and stalks. The resulting drugs might be consumed in forms other than pills and capsules. For example, you might smoke the dried leaves of one variety of people-plant hybrid to fight a cold, and for rich vitamin supplements you might garnish your salad with the leaves of another people-plant hybrid.

Clones, Clones, and More Clones

Cloning may turn out to be the fastest route to understanding genetic diseases, discovering the secrets of aging, and producing unlimited copies, not of ourselves, but of the tastiest, heartiest livestock. Cloning humans may one day be possible, but there is not a respected geneticist in the world who believes it has already been achieved.

In its broadest sense, cloning is asexual reproduction that results in a genetic duplicate of the original organism. Hundreds of organisms reproduce in this manner, and with plants such as orchids, cloning rare varieties is common. The "cloning boom" began in 1952, when two American biologists developed a technique whereby they substituted genetic material from one cell of an animal into the nucleus of an egg obtained from a female of the same species. Since then the "nuclear transfer" technique has been modified and refined, with the best success rate in cloning amphibians. Biologists have learned that in order to clone an organism, they must extract genetic material from the cells of a fetus or very young creature; adult cells, given the present state of the technology, can't be cloned. Yale biologist Dr. Clement Markert speculates that the nuclei of adult cells have become so specialized, or "irreversibly differentiated," that they have lost their flexibility to function as egg nuclei. (Incidentally, this is one of the major arguments geneticists have advanced to discredit David Rorvik's claim, in his controversial book *In His Image*, that a human has been successfully cloned: Rorvik's donor, millionaire "Max," is in his sixties.)

Cloning research is progressing on several fronts.

Mice from Tumors

To study specific genetic defects, Dr. Beatrice Mintz of the Fox Chase Institute for Cancer Research in Philadelphia is cloning mice to carry a single disease gene. Quite literally, Dr. Mintz turns a cancer cell into a living, normal-looking mouse, a feat

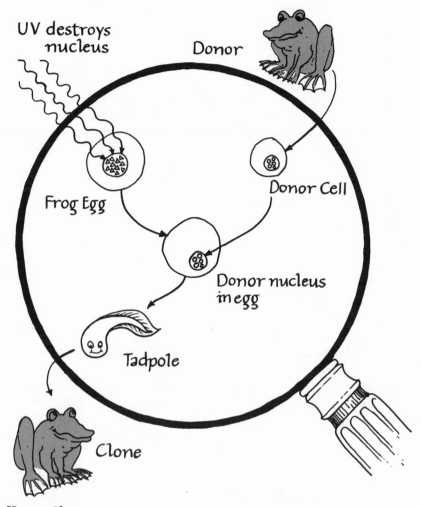

UV destroys nucleus

Donor

Frog Egg

Donor Cell

Donor nucleus in egg

Tadpole

Clone

How to Clone

Ultraviolet light is used to destroy the nucleus of a frog egg; that is, to destroy the mother's genetic material. A nucleus from a cell of the donor to be cloned (usually an intestine-cell nucleus) is inserted into the egg, which begins to divide and multiply, growing into a tadpole. Since the doctored egg contains genetic material from only the donor, the offspring has only one parent — itself — and is a true clone.

Gene Breakthroughs   83

that makes the alchemist's attempt to transmute lead into gold sound like child's play. To geneticists, Dr. Mintz's magic mice are gold: because they are grown from a diseased gene they are the living embodiment of that disease.

In one experiment she implanted in a tumor cell a gene believed to cause Lesch-Nyhan syndrome, a grotesque disorder in which young males develop such a compulsion to mutilate themselves that they often bite off their toes and lips. The altered tumor cells cloned themselves, and they were later injected into mouse embryos, which developed into adults whose offspring had Lesch-Nyhan disease. Such experiments provide geneticists with a unique opportunity to study the causes of disease and to attempt to design cures. Dr. Mintz has also demonstrated that not all mice whose "fathers" literally are cancer cells develop cancer. Many, in fact, grow to be perfectly healthy adults, which challenges the theory that malignant cells must be destroyed because they cannot be rehabilitated. Mintz is now trying to pinpoint the cellular process that she believes can, under certain conditions, transform malignant cells into healthy ones.

Prize Cows

Another gene alchemist is Yale's Dr. Markert. His current research could have a dramatic impact on animal husbandry in the coming decades. Whereas Dr. Mintz relies on diseased cells as the sires for her mice, Dr. Markert develops animals that have no fathers at all. He has been able to remove the male component of genes from an egg just fertilized, chemically stimulate the egg to divide, then reimplant the egg in a female mammal. The offspring herself (always a female) is not a clone, but because she bears no genetic male heritage, the eggs she produces as an adult exactly match her genes. If she were a prize-winning cow, for instance, then all her calves would deserve the same award. In other words, she can serve as the matriarch of a pure breed. Although only females can be produced by Markert's method, high-quality cows could be bred to prize bulls to guarantee Grade A herds. With this technique it might be possible to produce countless copies of prize dairy cows before the end of the century.

Human Clones

Will we ever be cloned? Many researchers assume it may eventually be possible, but wonder if there's anything to be gained from cloning humans. The diet and environment of a rat, rabbit, and even a cow can be carefully regulated to ensure that cloned offspring grow up like their parents. But if psychologists are right in their estimate that environment plays the major role in the development of human behavior and I.Q. (perhaps as much as 80 percent), then an infant who is a clone of his father, for example, could, as an adult, be as different from his father as if he had been conceived normally. Even a clone of Albert Einstein would not guarantee a genius. A cloned child could be endowed with a rich and pure genetic heritage, but the fate of that heritage would be shaped by countless uncontrollable factors.

8

Infertility Breakthroughs:
Children for Childless Couples

New hopes and cures for couples unable to have children will be in the forefront of medical advances in sexology during the 1980s. These treatments will be aimed at men as well as women, for it is becoming increasingly clear that husbands contribute to at least one third of all infertility problems.

Two of every ten couples can't have children. That number is expected to increase during the remainder of this century for several reasons. A rise in the number of abortions, an increase in venereal diseases, and the reliance on IUDs — all can cause uterine infection that, in turn, can scar and obstruct a woman's Fallopian tubes, making conception impossible. Another factor is that more and more women are postponing pregnancy to pursue careers, and a woman's reproductive capacity begins to decline in her mid twenties.

Where women once blamed themselves (and were blamed by their doctors) for barrenness in a marriage, recent findings indicate that men are often at fault. Too few sperm, sluggish sperm that peter out before reaching the egg, and sperm with deformed heads that can't penetrate an egg account for at least 15 percent of infertility complaints. Too much alcohol, certain antidepressant and anticancer drugs that act as toxins to the testes can also result in male infertility, as well as such simple factors as extremely tight underwear or a hot bath before sex. Another 8 percent of male infertility is due to infections and reversed vasectomies that scar and obstruct the ducts leading from the testes to the penis. Yet the most common cause of what some doctors refer to as "male barrenness" is the development of varicose veins in the scrotum, which can damage sperm, causing them to be either too weak or too maimed to fertilize an egg. The most recent estimates indicate that husbands account for as much as 40 percent of the infertility problems existing among couples. These insights into the causes of female and male barrenness are suggesting new cures for childless couples.

Help for Infertile Men
Clearing the Way for Obstructed Sperm

Improved surgical techniques will remedy this common problem. Several researchers are working to refine microsurgical techniques to clear scarred ducts and remove varicose veins from testes. Obstructions can now be easily detected by checking for impeded blood flow in the testes through use of the Doppler, or sounding, stethoscope. But Dr. Larry Lipshultz of the University of Texas Medical School in Houston says that present microsurgical techniques can open obstructed paths only if the problem is discovered early enough, before scarring becomes extensive. Finer surgical instruments connected to microscopes are also expected to help repair vasectomies, which can be reversed about 50 percent of the time; many men who undergo vasectomy-reversal surgery produce normal amounts of sperm, but for some unknown reason remain infertile. Some experts predict that by the end of the decade vasectomy-reversal surgery will be successful for about 80 percent of patients. Still, doctors caution that even with the most sophisticated surgical procedures, there may be a cut-off point — about ten years — after which vasectomies are probably irreversible. And if they could be reversed, fertility for some reason might never be fully restored. Researchers hope soon to understand this mystery.

Boosting the Sperm Count

Often a man does not produce a sufficient quantity of sperm to guarantee fertilization. Doctors believe that for fertilization to occur successfully a man should ideally produce between twenty million to sixty million sperm per milliliter of semen — about a thimbleful. Producing fewer does not necessarily indicate infertility, but the probability of a sperm-egg encounter drops; there is a lower limit (roughly four million sperm per milliliter), after which the probability of conception is almost zero. The number of sperm produced can in some cases be affected by the amount of sex hormones a man produces, and hormone production, in turn, may be affected by diet. At the University of Pittsburgh Hospital School of Medicine, Dr. Charles Cobb has uncovered evidence that the male hormone testosterone may be inhibited by too much alcohol. Alcoholics have long been known to suffer fertility loss, but many researchers assumed this to be a secondary effect of liver damage. Cobb has demonstrated, in rats at least, that moderate-to-large amounts of alcohol cut down the amount of testosterone and reduce sperm production. To help men with low sperm counts, researchers have begun testing various hormones on male volunteers. They anticipate that within a decade they will have developed either a pill or an injection to boost the sperm count in infertile men.

Improving the Health of Sperm

It takes healthy sperm to fight their way up the reproductive stream and bore through an egg's protective coating. Although a man may produce copious amounts of sperm each time he ejaculates, most sperm are often too weak to do the job. At the University of Rochester, Dr. Anthony Caldamone has accumulated preliminary evidence that lethargic, languid sperm may result partly from a dietary zinc deficiency. Dr. Caldamone has prescribed zinc tablets for infertile men, and in some instances fertility has been restored, though how the zinc works remains a mystery. Dr. Caldamone intends to continue his tests on infertile men to determine whether they may be deficient in other minerals or vitamins.

Compensating for Deformed Sperm

The shape of sperm may prove another important factor in determining whether a man is fertile or infertile. Sperm heads should be sharply oval, but in some infertile men the sperm are frequently characterized by round, blunt heads. Consequently, they literally bump into an egg rather than latch on to and penetrate it. In various men, deformities may result from exposure to environmental pollutants and radiation. Animal studies at the

National Institute of Child Health Development have shown that mice exposed to carcinogens produce abnormally bulbous and dented sperm that usually are incapable of fertilizing an egg. In the few cases where fertilization does occur, the embryo is soon aborted. According to researchers, this may indicate that abnormally shaped sperm contain defective genes resulting from environmental pollutants or congenital genetic flaws; there is strong evidence, for instance, that men with cystic fibrosis tend to produce oddly shaped sperm, a condition that is often responsible for infertility.

It appears that many infertile men produce their weakest or most deformed sperm at the end of each ejaculation and the most vital ones at the beginning. This observation may offer a cure for one form of infertility. Doctors have already registered initial success with infertile men by collecting only the sperm from the initial portion of the ejaculate and injecting them into the wife's cervix.

Yet before male infertility can be cured it must be diagnosed, and here there can be problems. One major difficulty, doctors assert, is that many men suspected of being infertile refuse to submit to sperm tests, feeling that a low sperm count, or deformed sperm, derogates their masculinity. There is no truth, of course, to that belief.

If, on the other hand, a man's infertility is due to genetically defective sperm, there is at present nothing that can be done to help. Treatment to correct genetically defective sperm lies at least twenty years in the future. (See *Gene Therapy*, p. 75.) However, for other kinds of infertility, refined microsurgical techniques are just around the corner.

Help for Infertile Women
Drugs to Encourage Ovulation

About 25 percent of female infertility is due to failure to ovulate. Many women fail to menstruate because their bodies secrete excessive amounts of the hormone prolactin, a condition known as hyperprolactinemia. Although it hasn't yet been determined how high prolactin concentrations in the blood inhibit ovulation, nor why so many women suffer from hyperprolactinemia, doctors are nevertheless working on new drugs to help infertile women ovulate.

Until a few years ago, the hormone HMG (human menopausal gonadotropin) — the first of the female fertility drugs — provided the single effective means for an infertile woman to become pregnant. But women faced a major hazard in taking HMG: it often made them too fertile. Many produced numerous eggs simultaneously and as a result often gave birth to as many as a half-dozen babies or more (though not all were viable). Today, the preferred fertility drug is Clomid (clomiphene citrate), but like HMG it too has drawbacks. Because it produces less ovarian stimulation than HMG, it diminishes the likelihood of multiple births, but for the same reason it reduces to 30 percent the number of women who can expect to become pregnant. A newer drug still being tested is LHRH (luteinizing-hormone releasing hormone). Because it acts on the pituitary gland, and only indirectly on the ovaries, scientists believe it should prevent overstimulation and multiple births. At Tulane University scientists have produced LHRH in two forms, a pill and a nasal spray, that have proven equally effective in tests; but like Clomid, LHRH offers an infertile woman only about a 30 percent chance of becoming pregnant. Tulane researchers, however, think the drug has greater potential than other fertility drugs and that they have just not yet figured out the optimum dose, or, perhaps, the most effective way to administer it.

The most promising new drug for women who fail to ovulate because they secrete too much prolactin may be Parlodel (bromocriptine mesylate); it binds to receptors in the pituitary gland and inhibits the production of prolactin. Parlodel — produced by the Swiss-based pharmaceutical company Sandoz — was approved by the FDA in August 1978 for the treatment of galactorrhea (the persistent flow of milk from the breasts) and for amenorrhea (the failure to menstruate), but not specifically for infertility. Still, many doctors prescribe Parlodel while they profess to be treating galactorrhea or amenorrhea. So long as the FDA does not formally label Parlodel a fertility drug, doctors will continue to avoid prescribing it for infertility for fear that they will be held responsible for any birth defects that might result.

Parlodel has been used for years in Europe, and there is no evidence that it causes birth defects. The FDA, however, feels that the European patients are too small a sample group adequately to prove the drug's safety. Tests with Parlodel are being conducted in the United States to determine whether it should be explicitly labeled a fertility drug, and a decision is expected by the mid 1980s. Since the drug is already on the market, if the tests prove positive, there would be no delay in doctors' being able to prescribe it for infertility problems.

Opening Tubes

About 40 percent of the cases of infertility in women are due to blocked Fallopian tubes. As with men, tubes can become blocked because of infection or voluntary sterilization. For some women, then, a new technique in microsurgery offers a solution. In a tedious four-hour operation a surgeon cuts and scrapes the obstructions from the tubes at three different layers and sews up the tubes one layer at a time. According to Dr. Richard Falk of the Columbia Hospital for Women in Washington, D.C., the best candidates for microsurgery are women who have been sterilized by having a section of their tubes looped out and tied, since this usually produces a clean break that can easily be mended. Dr. Falk claims that about 15 percent of the women who have been sterilized want the operation reversed, and for them microsurgery works about 75 percent of the time.

The worst candidates for microsurgery are women whose tubes have been scarred by infections, such as those caused by gonorrhea. These women have only a 20 percent chance of becoming pregnant, says Dr. Falk, and even if they do, it is likely that the embryo will embed itself in the tube, causing an ectopic pregnancy that can end in a rupture of the tube, a spontaneous abortion, and a life-threatening hemorrhage.

Although microsurgical techniques are bound to improve over the years, there are still many women with such extensive tube obstructions that no amount of surgery will help. There was a time when these women were doomed to remain childless, but the new breakthrough of *in vitro* fertilization pioneered by the British doctors Patrick Steptoe and Robert Edwards may soon remedy that.

Test-Tube Babies

The test-tube fertilization that resulted in the birth of Louise Brown on July 25, 1978, constituted an epochal event in medicine that may become commonplace within our lifetime. A few months later, on October 3, the world's second baby conceived in a test tube (really a circular glass Petri dish) was born in a Calcutta hospital in India, and in early 1979 a third baby was born in Scotland. Some gynecologists believe that by 1985 thousands of women with blocked Fallopian tubes (the condition Louise's mother suffered) will be pregnant through *in vitro* fertilization.

The fertilization techniques will not necessarily be similar. The egg removed surgically from Mrs. Brown — via a laparoscope inserted through a small incision in the abdomen — was united with sperm from her husband in a Petri dish and nurtured there for two and a half days before the tiny embryo was implanted in Mrs. Brown's uterus. The Indian doctors not only used a different approach, but advanced the technology of conception. Entering through the vagina, they made a small cut in the mother's ovary and gently withdrew ripened ova. The ova were fertilized in a Petri dish with the father's sperm, *but they were then stored in a deep freeze for fifty-three days before one embryo was thawed and implanted in the mother's uterus.* Thus, for almost two months, several potential human beings existed in a state of suspended animation.

The implications of this breakthrough are staggering. Infertile couples could conceive several children in a test tube at one time and then have the eggs frozen; whenever they wanted to have a child one egg could be thawed and implanted in the mother. How long could very young embryos be frozen before being safely thawed? Because the cells of a young embryo are so simple and similar in structure, doctors anticipate that fertilized eggs could be frozen for decades. (An extreme extension of this procedure involves an infant girl conceived *in vitro*. As an adult she could be implanted with an embryo produced by her parents, thus giving birth to her parents' child, her own genetic brother or sister.) Biologist Stanley Leibo of the Oak Ridge National Laboratory offers this fanciful though real possibility: "It is conceivable that an embryo that would otherwise develop into an adult in the 20th century could be frozen and stored close to [the temperature of] absolute zero for a millennium, to begin its life in the 30th century. The freezing of biological systems, then, offers the potential for the human being to control time, rather than the reverse." Dr. Steptoe predicts that during the 1980s several clinics will open around the world offering *in vitro* (literally "in glass") conception to infertile couples for under $1000. They may even offer to store your future children on ice.

No doubt moral, medical, and legal aspects of *in vitro* fertilization will be widely debated in this decade. Is a frozen fertilized egg a human being? Is destroying an embryo in a Petri dish — or simply discarding those embryos not transferred to the mother — a form of abortion? Does the technique of *in vitro* fertilization and the subsequent transfer of the embryo to the mother increase the risk of fetal abnormalities? Are researchers, doctors, hospitals, universities, or even government agencies that provide funding legally liable for abnormalities suffered by a child produced by *in vitro* techniques? And will the *in vitro* procedure culminate in selective breeding and wombs for hire? These are the questions that the recently formed Ethics Advisory Board of the Health, Education, and Welfare Department intends to resolve before *in vitro* fertilization becomes commonplace. They'll have to work fast. No doctor doubts that one day soon women with blocked Fallopian tubes and men with low sperm counts will eventually become parents through conception that takes place outside the mother's body.

What Next?

It is unlikely that scientists will be satisfied with stopping at *in vitro* fertilization. In fact they are already moving toward the next logical breakthrough: babies conceived in a test tube, and developed the full nine months in an artificial womb.

Several laboratories in the United States and England are recording slow but steady progress in *in vitro* gestation. Though the researchers are understandably reluctant to discuss their work at this early stage, they are experimenting with artificial wombs in hamsters, mice, and rabbits. There is no difficulty in fertilizing an egg, inducing it through several healthy cell divisions, or in feeding the *in vitro* embryo a balance of nutrients for several days or weeks. The immense problem that no one has yet solved — and probably won't for many years — is how to provide an ample supply of oxygenated blood to the fetus and to remove wastes from the life-supporting bath surrounding the fetus. These are functions normally handled by a mother's kidneys, liver, and blood stream.

The artificial womb and its backup systems must, of course, be fail-safe, performing perfectly for nine months. As large as that problem is, it's not insurmountable. During the 1980s and 1990s scientists are expected to make major improvements in artificial kidneys, livers, hearts, and blood-filtering systems — and each advance will augur further progress toward the perfect artificial womb. Since the diet of a fetus in an artificial womb can be carefully controlled, researchers believe that these wombs will ultimately prove to be more beneficial environments for fetuses than a mother's womb. Also, artificial wombs will enable doctors more easily to scrutinize a developing embryo for abnormalities.

Despite the medical complexities, legal snafus, and moral outcries that *in vitro* gestation will surely engender, many scientists claim that the successful creation of an artificial womb will occur in the first half of the next century. The initial human tests will surely be performed in secrecy — as were early *in vitro* fertilization experiments. Researchers in the field are bound to emphasize the many advantages of *in vitro* gestation: it's easy and painless; parents will be able to visit their growing child, watch it take human form, kick, and suck its thumb; and at a time convenient to doctor and parents the hatch will be opened and the baby born gently, effortlessly. Actually witnessing the development of your child should prove to be an awesome experience. How this phenomenon and the complex moral and social issues surrounding it will affect the parents of the twenty-first century remains to be examined. But given our proclivities for increased leisure time, greater convenience, and full equality between the sexes, *in vitro* gestation is bound to catch on. And big.

9

Female Health Breakthroughs:
Medicine for Wives, Mothers, and Working Women

Diseases of the Liberated Woman

If you're a "liberated" woman, chances are you're contracting diseases and developing ailments that were once exclusive to men. In fact, doctors foresee major changes over the next two decades in women's health and longevity. Liberation is being won at a price.

Women today outlive men by an average of 5.7 years. Traditionally, women have not been very susceptible to ulcers and diseases of the lungs, and apparently from adolescence through menopause the hormone estrogen provides them with built-in protection against many kinds of heart disease. Yet in the last few years women's lead in health — and possibly in longevity — has begun to slip. According to a national study, the number of women suffering from peptic ulcers — long regarded a male disease — is up 13 percent. Up also are women's blood pressure levels, the incidence of emphysema, and lung cancer. And Dr. Theodore Cooper, former director of the National Heart and Lung Institute, claims that 11 percent more women under the age of forty-five suffer heart attacks than was true several years ago. The American Cancer Society predicts that by the end of this century as many women smokers will die from lung cancer as men.

Contemporary women are also experiencing an increase in psychological disorders. The number of women admitted to public and private psychiatric hospitals since 1970 has almost doubled, and in this period the female suicide rate has risen. In 1977 the National Institute on Drug Abuse released these statistics: forty-seven million American women take tranquilizers and sedatives (compared with twenty-nine million men), twelve million women use stimulants daily (compared with five million men), and approximately five million women are now alcoholics.

Before the year 2000, some authorities speculate that women could lose their lead in longevity. "The women's liberation movement has opened up new options for women," says Dr. Kenneth Greenspan of Columbia University's Physicians and Surgeons. "Grappling with these options and the challenges they present can be extremely debilitating." Even many of the women who choose to stay at home are suffering, according to New York psychiatrist Dr. Alexandra Symonds, because they feel less productive in the home and experience chronic guilt over being considered second-class citizens.

No two people, of course, react to stress in the same manner. Many women thrive on the challenges their careers offer. Nonetheless, these women, too, are experiencing changes in their health. It is important for you to know what to expect in the next ten to twenty years.

Who Copes Better — Women or Men?

Do women have a biological handicap in coping with stress, or has nature endowed them with an advantage — one that has lain dormant throughout their years of oppression? If so, can this advantage be realized? These are a cross-section of the topics that stress specialists will examine during the 1980s.

Scientists believe that in our evolutionary past men were expendable at an early age — to be precise, after they impregnated one or more women. Women, though, were required to live longer in order to rear children, so nature endowed them with the protective hormone estrogen. If this capsule summary were accurate, then women should be genetically healthier than men. However, recent studies suggest that women in fiercely competitive jobs, who are forced to adopt highly aggressive behavior, lose the advantage of estrogen. This factor may be a substantial cause for the increase in heart disease among women. Some scientists wonder whether estrogen eventually will completely lose its effectiveness in warding off heart problems.

Although men under extreme stress most often develop ulcers and heart attacks, women in stressful situations are generally more susceptible to a host of sexual disorders, ranging from frigidity to painful intercourse and menstruation. Problems of water retention, irregular menstruation, and decreased milk secretion — which can affect breast-feeding — have also recently been implicated in the female stress-illness link. Rheumatoid arthritis is another stress-related disease peculiar to women: four out of five victims are women who are unhappy with the traditional female sex-career roles but feel too helpless to improve their situation. There is slight evidence, not yet conclusive, that urinogenital cancer in women is stress-related.

A woman's physiological responses to stressful demands vary considerably from a man's. Dr. Marianne Frankenhaeuser of the University of Stockholm investigated the effects of stress on workers by measuring certain chemical indicators of stress in their urine. During pleasant, nonstressful situations men and women produced the same amounts of adrenalines (adjusting for body weight). Yet when the groups were compared while taking intelligence tests under time pressure, men produced far more of the coping chemicals than women.

Still, too little is known about the physiology of stress in women to conclude that men are biologically better equipped to handle stress. Dr. Frankenhaeuser believes women may have a completely different and as-yet-undetected hormonal mechanism for coping with stress — perhaps more effective than a man's. Or that the response to stress may be a learned pattern, and as more women are exposed to increasingly stressful situations, their bodies will learn to produce greater quantities of adrenalines.

Women are becoming the focus of intensive health research. It is almost certain that as we move through the 1980s, statistics relating to women's health will be grimmer. But with stepped-up research, scientists may discover drugs, behavioral therapies, and biofeedback techniques to lighten the burden of stress, not only for women, but also for men, who themselves don't cope all that well with the stress of modern living.

An Injection to Prevent Pregnancy

A simple shot in the arm or buttock may soon offer immunization against pregnancy. American scientists expect to begin clinical tests of a pregnancy vaccine by 1982, and if trials run smoothly, the drug could be on the market by the mid-to-late 1980s. The vaccine will offer women immunity to pregnancy by nullifying the effect of a specific hormone essential for reproduction.

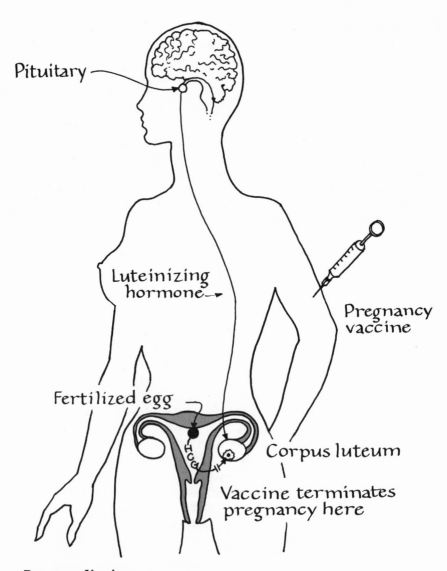

Pituitary

Luteinizing hormone—►

Pregnancy vaccine

Fertilized egg

Corpus luteum

Vaccine terminates pregnancy here

Pregnancy Vaccine

The pituitary gland releases luteinizing hormone, which stimulates the corpus luteum to produce progesterone, the hormone needed to prepare the woman's body for pregnancy. If the egg is not fertilized, progesterone levels fall and menstrual bleeding occurs. If the egg is fertilized, it releases human chorionic gonadotropin (HCG), which encourages the corpus luteum to continue secreting vital progesterone. The pregnancy vaccine would block the action of HCG, thus terminating pregnancy because of the absence of progesterone.

The hormone, human chorionic gonadotropin (HCG), is synthesized in the woman's body six to eight days after fertilization of the egg. This hormone permits the development of the corpus luteum, a vital substance formed in the ovary immediately after ovulation. Without HCG, the corpus luteum sloughs off in menstruation. Since HCG has to travel through the blood stream to reach the ovaries, it should be an easy, and ideal, target to capture and destroy with antibodies planted in the circulatory system; in other words, with a vaccine. The trick has been to create the right vaccine to prevent HCG from reaching the ovaries every time an egg is fertilized.

In 1971, Dr. Vernon Stevens of the Department of Obstetrics and Gynecology of Ohio State University was the first scientist to demonstrate through experiments with baboons that pregnancy could be prevented by blocking the HCG hormone. Since then, scientists at the Merck Institute for Therapeutic Research have successfully immunized female hamsters and rabbits against pregnancy. None of the animals has experienced any ill effects from immunization, and all of them have subsequently regained complete fertility. Such reversibility, of course, is one of the main requirements of any human pregnancy vaccine.

Similar experiments have also been performed on women by biochemist G. P. Talwar at the All-India Institute of Medical Science. In the mid 1970s, Dr. Talwar successfully immunized several women against pregnancy for up to a year, during which time most of them experienced normal menstruation. After the effect of the immunization wore off, two of the women successfully gave birth. But the vaccine Dr. Talwar developed worked only some of the time and often produced unpleasant side effects. In 1978 he abandoned these tests to return to animal studies.

While Dr. Talwar is trying to perfect his vaccine, Dr. Stevens thinks he's produced one that's ready for clinical tests. Dr. Stevens' vaccine captures HCG and inactivates it without interfering with other hormones in the body. Eventually, of course, its effect wears off. Working with scientists from three major drug companies, Dr. Stevens plans to vaccinate healthy fertile volunteers as early as 1982. If he's right, none of them should have to worry about becoming pregnant for quite a while.

By the late 1980s women may be able to select from vaccines with various immunization periods; for one year, for example, or perhaps up to five years.

The Do-It-Yourself Pregnancy Test

If the antipregnancy test should occasionally fail to work, at least the woman will be able quickly to determine in the privacy of her own bedroom whether she's pregnant.

A pregnancy-detection package labeled E.P.T. (Early Pregnancy Test) is already available in drugstores in some states without a prescription and sells for less than $10. The device operates by detecting that vital pregnancy hormone HCG, which is eliminated in the urine as early as the ninth day after the first menstrual period is missed. According to the manufacturers, a positive reaction to the test indicates a 97 percent certainty of pregnancy.

The test is quick and simple. A morning's sample of urine (which contains more HCG than samples taken later in the day) is mixed with purified water and a package of special chemicals. The mixture is then shaken for ten seconds and allowed to stand for two hours. A dark brown ring in the bottom of the test tube indicates that the pregnancy hormone is present in your urine. If the hormone is not present, a yellow-red stain is visible, and this negative result is about 80 percent accurate. If menstruation doesn't begin within a week, you can perform a second test, which has an improved accuracy of 91 percent.

A fast, nonprescription test offers benefits other than the advantage of an early abortion, if a woman elects that course. Also, since the first sixty days of pregnancy are among the most crucial in the development of the embryo, a very early diagnosis of pregnancy can help the mother guard against the hazards of alcohol and drugs, smoking, and improper nutrition. The simple test, which by the mid 1980s should be available everywhere in the United States, should be particularly comforting for women who have irregular periods and must anxiously wait to learn if this time they're *really* pregnant.

Do-It-Yourself Abortions

If a woman in the 1980s is pregnant and decides to have an abortion, she'll be able to induce one safely.

British researchers at the John Radcliffe Hospital have tested a self-inducing abortion device on more than 200 women and report excellent results. The device consists of a vaginal pessary that contains a chemical which in a matter of hours induces contractions that abort the fetus. All of the women tested considered the pessary easy to insert and comfortable to wear, and British doctors claim that in 83 percent of the cases pregnancy terminated quickly and with virtually no unwarranted side effects. The minor nausea and cramps a few of the women reported lasted only four to eight hours. The pessary has been used only under medical supervision, and even when the device is commercially available, such abortions may be performed in a hospital or gynecologist's office because of the slight risk of hemorrhage. Women who have worn the pessary thus far have been no more than twenty days pregnant. Radcliffe doctors still haven't determined just how many weeks into a pregnancy a woman could still safely use the pessary.

The advantages of the new device are both physical and psychological. If a woman suspects she's pregnant, by using the pessary she could avoid the delay in waiting for a positive diagnosis. In addition, she eliminates the emotional stress involved in a surgical abortion. In their medical report, the Radcliffe doctors write: "There is little doubt that the interruption of very early pregnancy, before major embryological developments have taken place, is much more acceptable physically, emotionally, and psychologically." Research on the pessary is being sponsored by the World Health Organization, which hopes eventually to introduce the device into Third World countries burdened with soaring birth rates. The Radcliffe doctors say they need a few more years of testing before they'll be completely satisfed with the technique, but they are fairly certain that the abortion device could be available from most gynecologists by the mid 1980s.

Part II

Science

10

Biorhythm Breakthroughs:
New Rhythms That Make You Tick

Resetting Your Master Clock

On a flight from New York to Greece, as you pass over Barcelona, you take a yellow and blue capsule so that when you land in Athens you won't experience jet lag. The capsule is not an "upper": you're not racing, and you'll not be doubly exhausted when its effect wears off. The capsule resets your twenty-four-hour biological clock — hormonal secretions, temperature fluctuations, sleep-wake cycles. Everything has been precisely adjusted.

A wealth of scientific evidence documents the effects of biological rhythms on sleeping, waking, hunger, sexual arousal and moods, physical and mental alertness, and even on animal's and man's vulnerability to drugs and toxins. Mice, for example, fed a carcinogenic diet at one time of day develop more tumors than mice fed the same diet a few hours later. Skin grafts on hamsters have less chance of being rejected if performed before late afternoon, when the animal's biological clock raises body temperature. Time-grafting studies are now underway on humans. Doctors have already learned that heart patients are most sensitive to digitalis, and diabetics to insulin, between four to seven in the morning. So dramatic, in fact, are the time-related effects of drugs that many hospitals administer chemotherapy to cancer patients synchronized with certain biorhythms.

There is a biological clock that times your life's rhythms; it may also be the master timekeeper of the clock that governs aging. Locating it is one of the greatest challenges facing modern biology. Dr. Robert Moore of the University of California at La Jolla has come about as close as any scientist to pinpointing its location in our bodies. He is "99 percent" sure that the clock consists of a tiny cluster of neurons, at the base of the brain, called the suprachiasmatic nucleus. When this neuron cluster is destroyed by electrodes in rats and hamsters, many of their major hormonal rhythms disappear, disrupting sleep and waking, metabolism and sexual cycles. Moore still needs objective proof that the suprachiasmatic nucleus performs the same function in people, but he's encouraged by the fact that the neuron cluster "is in precisely the same location in humans that it is in the animals studied, and it has the same appearance."

Biorhythm Bonanza

An understanding of the mechanisms of this master clock could yield many practical breakthroughs. Some psychologists believe that personality and I.Q. tests may produce significantly different results depending on the time of day they are taken. In fact, certain psychiatric illnesses categorized as "affective disorders" — including manic-depressive psychosis, depression, and involutional melancholia — may be due to desynchronized biorhythms. Interestingly enough, such common maladies as insomnia, loss of appetite, and sexual dysfunctions can often be cured by resetting the biological clock. NASA biologists say that until they determine how biorhythms affect mood, attentiveness, and efficiency, they cannot confidently launch the era of long-distance manned space travel; astronauts could easily be mentally and physically wiped out by whopping jet lags.

Solving the clock riddle also ought to settle many popular claims made for biorhythms. Do we really have twenty-three-day physical cycles, twenty-eight-day emotional cycles, and thirty-three-day intellectual cycles? Are we accident prone when our cycles switch from plus to minus? Why do both homicides and admissions to psychiatric hospitals seem to peak at full moon and new moon?

Your Daily Biopeaks

You may one day plan your professional and personal life to make optimum use of particular biological cycles. Facts emerging from biorhythm research are beginning to hint at how this may be done, and they dramatically demonstrate how much of daily life is influenced — if not governed — by the ticking of your biological clock.

Midnight to 4:00 A.M.	Most of your body functions are at their lowest ebb, but your hearing is at its sharpest (a fact not commonly appreciated by burglars). You shouldn't be surprised; prehistoric man relied on this radar to protect him while he slept.
7:00 A.M.	Your adrenal hormones peak, your heart rate increases, your body temperature rises, and blood pulses more strongly through your body. Nature's own alarm.
8:00 A.M.	Your sex-hormone production is at a peak (not at the traditional romantic hour of dusk). Men are more aware of this than women.
9:00 A.M.	Grease splashes from the frying pan and you flinch a bit. You drink hot coffee without any discomfort. At this hour your body is least sensitive to pain. It may be your brain's peak time for production of its own opiates, the enkephalins and endorphins; a time when painkilling drugs are least needed.
10:00 A.M.	If you're introverted, your concentration and memory for acquiring new facts peak. Your work efficiency is highest at this time. (Extroverts, you must wait.)
Noon	Your body's most susceptible to the effects of alcohol. That's why a martini lunch can be disastrous to your performance for the rest of the day.
2:00 P.M.	Almost everyone experiences a postlunch energy dip. It has less to do with what you've eaten than with your normal midday hormonal changes.
3:00 P.M.	Extroverts are at their analytical and creative prime, and will be for several hours. Introverts are coming off their peak.
4:00 P.M.	Flushed? Perspiring? Breathing heavily? It's due to changes in your body metabolism as it gears up for the second half of the day.

5:00 P.M.	Your senses of smell and taste are most acute (a dangerous time for weight watchers). Your hearing has attained its second daily peak.
6:00 P.M.	Ironically, when most of us are sitting on commuter trains, buses, or in our cars, our potential for physical activity is at its peak. Strength and stamina have reached a daily high, though psychological factors can sap this energy.
7:00 P.M.	Your temper and irritability can flare because of hormonal changes; your blood pressure peaks and emotions are shakiest.
8:00 P.M.	The day's food and water have been stored, so the body's weight has reached its maximum (the wrong time to step on a scale).
10:00 P.M.	The blahs? Your hormone levels and body temperatures are down; breathing slows; your body is at an overall performance low.
Midnight	Your body begins its hardest work, replacing dead cells and building new cells for the next day.

Your I.Q. Rhythm

Genes and environment contribute their share (as yet undetermined) to intelligence. But a third factor that may play a role in your I.Q. could be an unsuspected biorhythm between nerve cells in your brain.

University of California psychologist Arthur Jensen stirred controversy in 1969 when he argued that genetic factors are more important than environmental ones in influencing I.Q. After testing Southern blacks in 1977, Jensen modified his ideas somewhat to acknowledge the importance of environment. Since then he believes he has discovered another measure of intelligence, based on a person's reaction time. He studied more than 400 university and vocational students, grade-schoolers, and the mentally retarded. Using a panel of colored lights with buttons beneath them, he measured how fast a person could dart his finger from one button to another in chasing the flashing lights. The task is clocked in thousandths of a second and is so simple that your reaction occurs faster than your thoughts. Jensen found that the reaction times of all his subjects correlated with their scores on I.Q. tests: the higher a person's I.Q., the faster the reaction time.

"This shows that mental ability measured by standard intelligence tests is getting at something much more basic than skills acquired at school or home, or than specific knowledge," he says. That basic something, Jensen suspects, is a personal "rhythm" between nerve cells in the brain. The faster your neural rhythm, the better the chance for switched-on cells to relay information — thus, the greater your intelligence.

Does this mean that all athletes, renowned for their fast reaction time, are the smartest people? Apparently not. Jensen says his test measures a different and more fundamental reaction time, and that Muhammad Ali, for instance, tested by a procedure similar to Jensen's buttons and lights, scored no better than the average college student. Jensen has been controversial for more than a decade, and although he has softened his genetic views, his new work guarantees he'll remain in the hot spotlight. In his reaction-time tests, university students scored higher than vocational college students, the retarded scored lowest, and blacks slightly lower than whites.

Other psychologists have begun to test Jensen's hypothesis between reaction time and I.Q. If he is proved right, your children, in addition to taking college boards, may have to score high on reaction-time tests to gain admission to college. And where the accuracy of present I.Q. tests has been challenged as being biased against people of certain social and ethnic backgrounds, reaction-time tests, which involve only pressing buttons, could not be similarly criticized. In fact, these tests may turn out to be the only totally impartial and fair I.Q. tests educators will ever have.

Time Therapy for Insomniacs

For insomniacs who suffer from biological clocks that are out of sync with their environment, help is coming in the way of chronotherapy. (*Chronos* is the Greek word for time.) Two major sleep centers are reporting good results in shifting faulty biorhythms, and this time therapy could become a standard treatment in a few years. Best of all, you can safely administer it to yourself at home.

Insomniacs' problems are not always psychological; they may be unsuspecting victims of shifted biological rhythms. Instead of running on a twenty-four-hour cycle of hormonal secretions and temperature highs and lows, they may run on cycles anywhere from twenty to twenty-eight hours. Even an hour's difference can be devastating. One day, for example, your body may naturally want to sleep from 11:00 P.M. to 7:00 A.M., the next day from 12:00 midnight to 8:00 A.M., the following day from 1:00 A.M. to 9:00 A.M., and so on. A sort of daily jet lag. This pattern has been recently diagnosed at several sleep clinics, and somnologists — scientists who study sleep — are surprised to find that the problem is not all that rare. "These people suffer from what we call phase-shifted dysomnia," says Dr. Charles Pollak of New York's Montefiore Sleep-Wake Disorder Unit in the Bronx. Pollak has reset the clocks of more than twenty-five insomniacs to tick in harmony with the rest of society.

Chronotherapy is also being tested at the Stanford University Sleep Clinic. The step-by-step technique is quite simple. If you usually fall asleep at 4:00 A.M., you're asked to go to sleep at 3:00 A.M. for a few nights. Once you've adapted to the shift, you move your bedtime back to 2:00 A.M., and so on.

The reason for human circadian rhythms that differ from the twenty-four-hour cycle is not understood, but it can cause serious problems with married people. At the Family Studies Center of the University of Missouri in Kansas City, researchers examined the impact of mismatched bio-cycles on twenty-eight married couples. They concluded that when an "owl" is married to a "lark," the couple share fewer activities, have fewer sexual encounters, engage in fewer serious conversations, have more unresolved conflicts, and run a far greater risk of divorce. They also found that family life can be thrown into disarray if a child's biological clock does not tick in time with his parents.

How can you determine if your sleeplessness is the result of phase-shifted dysomnia? The diagnosis can easily be done at home. Pollak suggests keeping a log of your preferred bedtimes. If you find that you're not sleepy at 11:00 P.M., but always at four in the morning, or if your preferred bedtime over any given month slides round the clock, then your biological ticker is out of sync. Pollak claims that since most general physicians aren't aware of the prevalence of phase-shifted dysomnia, they treat the problem by suggesting such sure-to-fail remedies as reading a dull book, drinking warm milk, or, worst of all, by prescribing sleeping pills that only aggravate the condition.

Depression and Your Faulty Clock

We all experience highs and lows in our moods, but if those swings are strong enough, and frequent enough, they can constitute debilitating illnesses — mania, depression, or the commingled manic-depressive psychosis. There is growing evidence that these affective disorders, plaguing one out of ten Americans, are caused by biological clocks with cycles slightly longer or shorter than the normal twenty-four hours. A promising cure — at least as effective as drugs — may be chronotherapy.

The most illuminating research on the biorhythms underlying affective disorders has been conducted at the National Institute of Mental Health's Clinical Psychobiology Branch in Bethesda, Maryland. In 1978, NIMH psychiatrists closely monitored many depressive and manic-depressive patients. Each patient wore a motion-sensitive device around her or his wrist that traced all activities, day and night, waking and sleeping. The patients' blood was frequently analyzed for hormonal changes. A computer digested the data and printed out the chemical and physical highs and lows, and wake-sleep cycles. Instead of falling randomly, as it was long thought they did, the fluctuations traced out definite rhythms — ones that differed slightly from a normal person's circadian rhythms.

In manic-depressive patients the researchers learned that a few days before the manic phase set in, many patients would go to bed and wake up earlier than usual. By advancing the patients' bedtimes several hours, Dr. Frederick Goodwin, chief of psychobiology at the NIMH, was able to cure many patients of all their symptoms for about two weeks. Advancing their bedtimes again resulted in another two-week cure, but the effect could not be repeated a third time, perhaps, Goodwin believes, because three such changes returned the hands of the faulty clock back to their original abnormal positions. For some patients chronotherapy was as effective as drugs in alleviating their symptoms. Goodwin speculates that "maybe people (with affective disorders) are awake when they are supposed to be asleep."

Why did the cures last only two weeks? No one is exactly sure, but "two weeks is a very curious time," says Goodwin, pointing out that it also requires two weeks after the first dose for tricyclic and lithium drugs, used to treat affective disorders, to take effect.

Seasonal Cycles

Abnormal daily biorhythms may reveal only half the tale of mental illness: faulty seasonal or yearly patterns may also figure in this nightmare. In 1978 another team of NIMH scientists studied hormones in the blood of normal people over a year's time. They found that in January and July the brain's production of norepinephrine, a protein known to influence depression, hits a high, and the production of serotonin, the brain protein known for its tranquilizing effects, falls to a low. A few months later, in May and October, the opposite cycle occurs. Goodman hasn't yet concluded whether his patients are subject to abnormal yearly cycles, too, though that's a real possibility, since the new NIMH experiments have dramatized a clear daily distinction in norepinephrine production between normal and mentally ill people. In the normal group norepinephrine production in the brain peaks just before dawn and ends abruptly by daylight, but the peak in the manic patients occurs much earlier in the night, is stronger, and begins to ebb well before sunrise.

"We have to be very careful because all of this can sound like astrology," Goodwin cautions. "But cyclicity in human behavior is a real phenomenon that has been overlooked for too long." Goodwin hopes that within a few years his research on biorhythms will explain why certain drugs seem to work best when administered at a particular phase of a mental illness, or at a certain time of the year.

11

Brain Breakthroughs:
Your Body's Own Drugs for Pleasure and Pain

Crossing the street, you spot a berserk car aiming straight for you. This frightening image impinges on your brain's visual center, rushes to the seat of emotions, where it registers fear, then speeds to the motor controls that propel you to run. Image, emotion, action. A complete, complex mental event.

Fifty years ago, Sigmund Freud predicted that every mental event would one day be traced to chemical reactions in the brain. Today, scientists are proving him right. Not that their 1960s' analogy of the brain as a complex computer is wrong, but scientists are learning that a more fundamental and fruitful approach to understanding the brain's functions is to view it as a giant chemistry set. For the first time scientists are measuring minuscule amounts of brain chemicals, tagging them, and tracing their intricate pathways. Memory, concentration, fear — even aggression — have all recently been identified as chemical events. This fresh insight into the brain promises to yield major breakthroughs during the next two decades in the treatment of mental illness and the alleviation of pain. It also offers the possibility of increased creative ability. Here are several advances we can expect.

A Nasal Spray to Enhance Your Memory

Forgotten where you parked your car? Can't remember where you left your best dress to be altered? Sniff vasopressin and you'll remember.

Vasopressin is a hormone located in the cherry-sized pituitary gland, at the base of the brain. Scientists working with vasopressin have found that a few whiffs of the chemical can stimulate memory, even in the severest cases of amnesia and senility. What's more, the results are lasting. Vasopressin must be inhaled rather than taken orally because it is a member of the peptide family of organic compounds, which decompose in the digestive tract.

Recently, at the University of Liège in Belgium,, vasopressin experiments were conducted on a group of males between the ages of fifty and sixty-five. After receiving three doses of vasopressin for three consecutive days, the men registered significant improvement on memory and learning tests. In fact, one man who had remembered nothing for three months, from the time an auto accident left him in a fifteen-day coma, regained his full recall faculties on the seventh day of vasopressin treatment. In another experiment at Madrid's Hospital Clinico de San Carlos, doctors had similar success with the spray. Four amnesia patients, three suffering memory loss from car accidents and one from alcoholism, were treated with vasopressin, and within five days their amnesia disappeared.

Specifically how vasopressin works remains a mystery. First synthesized in 1968, the substance was initially known to help regulate the body's water content. The idea that vasopressin might affect memory was proposed by Dr. D. de Wied, a Dutch scientist at the University of Utrecht. Dr. de Wied discovered that by removing the pituitary gland in rats he could impair their memory and interfere with their learning ability. Identification of the hormone, and follow-up work with more rats, confirmed the link between vasopressin and memory: rats that sniffed vasopressin not only learned faster, but better remembered the paths through intricate mazes.

Vasopressin does produce mild side effects; namely, more rapid heartbeat and higher blood pressure, both of which can be potential problems, particularly for the elderly. But researchers assert that any undesirable effects may be eliminated without reducing vasopressin's effectiveness if the drug is administered in very small doses over longer periods of time. Sandoz, the company that synthesized the chemical, predicts it could market a completely safe version of vasopressin by 1985.

Thus far the hormone has been tested only on short-term memory — the ability to recall events of the recent past. But tests are underway to determine if vasopressin can also activate childhood memories, or possibly even help a person regain the facility with a foreign language learned earlier in life. Since vasopressin has already been prescribed in the treatment of diabetes, rigorous testing on people to document its effects on long-term memory should not take long. For the moment, though, vasopressin will be used primarily to treat amnesia victims. But in the near future, vasopressin may help you sharpen your memory and enhance your learning ability. The regular use of vasopressin may even sustain your brain's memory mechanism so that you could be spared the forgetfulness which usually accompanies old age.

Increasing Your Attention Span

The degree to which you can concentrate on a task may make the difference between success or failure. Some of us seem to be plagued by frustratingly short attention spans, which cause us to be easily distracted. If that's the problem, a shot of ACTH/MSH may offer a solution.

Amphetamines, the popular pep pills, speed up the mind, but they don't give it focused direction. There is, however, a natural brain protein that does both. It's present in two hormones located in the pituitary gland. One of these chemicals, ACTH (adrenocorticotropic hormone), is known to stimulate the secretion of sex hormones; the other, MSH (melanocyte-stimulating hormone), regulates the amount of dark brown pigment (melanin) in your skin. This "sex-tanning" compound may prove to be a chemical wonder.

In 1971, studies on rats showed that the ACTH/MSH protein improved memory. More recently, work by endocrinologist Dr. Abba Kastin of the Tulane University School of Medicine reveals that the protein produces a dual effect in people: it improves visual retention and heightens their powers of concentration. Students injected with the compound were better able to remember geometrical figures flashed before them, as well as to concentrate more effectively on their studies, and for longer periods of time. When the students' concentration was tested by a series of monotonous, repetitious tasks, those who received the brain protein scored higher than those injected with a placebo. It's possible that if you're one of those fortunate people who can concentrate despite the most tempting distractions, your body may naturally produce a generous amount of ACTH/MSH.

Perhaps the most significant discovery concerning ACTH/MSH is that it appears to be the only significant drug for the mentally retarded. Retarded patients given injections of the protein have been able to comprehend tasks more rapidly and demonstrate clearer thinking. This fact may indicate that some forms of retardation are caused by lack of a "concentration" compound. Also, Dr. Kastin has begun testing his hypothesis that ACTH/MSH may be effective in treating senile patients and hyperactive children. Certain forms of learning disabilities and senility may prove to be due to nothing more than the loss or congenital lack of sufficient amounts of the concentration hormone.

Relief from Anxiety and Aggression

Is aggressive behavior programed into our genes? Sociobiologists answer yes, behaviorists, no. The definite answer may not be decided for many years, but in the meantime, neurobiologists are clearly demonstrating that aggression has a chemical basis — and that violent behavior can be controlled by a balance of the brain's own chemicals.

Messages are routed through the brain by neurotransmitters — the chemicals that relay information from one nerve cell to another. (Until a few years ago, scientists thought there existed only a few major neurotransmitters. Today, however, they count over thirty and suspect dozens more will be discovered.) In 1978, in the first study of its kind with people, scientists at the National Institute of Mental Health found that human aggression appears to be regulated by two neurotransmitters, serotonin and norepinephrine. The tests were conducted by Dr. Frederick Goodwin of the NIMH on a group of navy enlisted men who had difficulty adjusting to military life. Through his research, Goodwin learned that those men with more serotonin in their spinal fluid scored lowest on aggression tests, but those with more norepinephrine scored highest. Goodwin's tests confirmed what earlier animal studies had suggested: a link between the two chemicals and aggressive behavior.

Goodwin and other scientists believe that any chemical controlling violent behavior works by suppressing either our primitive "reptilian" brain, which governs ritualistic and hierarchical aspects of life, or the more relatively recently evolved "limbic" brain, which governs our emotions and altruistic feelings. Anti-anxiety drugs, which have been administered time and again to dozens of species of animals, have invariably produced calming effects, and there is growing evidence that behavior-controlling drugs operate primarily on those sections of the human brain that evolved earliest.

Goodwin believes, however, that the neurotransmitter-aggression link isn't necessarily genetic. "One's environment, particularly early life experiences," he says, "can have an influence on biochemical balance." This may mean that a child repeatedly confronted with situations arousing aggressive behavior may learn to produce high levels of norepinephrine and low levels of serotonin — a pattern that remains throughout his life. According to Goodwin, there is a chemical available to correct the neurotransmitter imbalance. Lithium, which boosts serotonin levels in animals and makes them docile, has produced beneficial effects in recent tests on aggressive prisoners. Ethical issues, says Goodwin, are the only considerations that prevent immediate application of his findings.

A Pill for Your Fears

Are you afraid of heights, enclosures, strangers? Each of these fears, and other bothersome anxieties, may originate from specific molecules in the body. If these molecules could be chemically identified, your particular phobia could be cured by a drug.

Animal studies point to the possible existence of behavioral brain molecules. One such molecule may be a fear peptide, a tiny string of fifteen amino acids. In controversial tests, scientists at Houston's Baylor University College of Medicine and the University of Tennessee trained rats to fear the dark before killing them to extract various chemicals from their brains. One extract, every time it was injected into the brains of untrained rats, caused the animals to experience intense fear of the dark for a week. The scientists named this brain protein scotophobin, meaning "fear of the dark." What surprised them even more than the rats' reaction was their subsequent observation that when modified rat scotophobin was injected into goldfish, the fish stayed in the open during daylight hours. The goldfish wouldn't even venture into the shadow of a rock for food!

The results of the scotophobin experiments have been doubted by many scientists who claim that this research does not prove that learned behavior can be so neatly contained in a chemical and then transferred from one creature to another. But in 1978, German scientists, working with honey bees, demonstrated that at least another type of learned behavior, "time sense," appears to reside in a molecule and can be transmitted from one bee to another. At Würzburg's Zoologisches Institut scientists trained bees to feed from a bowl of sugar water at a set time each day. Brain tissue from these insects was then surgically inserted into spaces on both sides of the brains of other bees. For two days the recipients showed no special feeding pattern. But on the third day — and for only that one day — 60 percent of the bees suddenly fed at exactly the donors' preferred time. The scientists found no evidence that nerve connections had formed between graft and brain, and concluded that the donor bees' learned time sense was most likely chemically transferred to the recipients, and that the messages were probably too weak to dominate the recipients' behavior for more than a short time.

Neuroscientists have reason to believe that the chemicals governing such animal "emotions" as fear, loyalty, and hostility may not be substantially different from those chemicals yet to be isolated in people. Some time within the next two decades a chemical model of the brain should provide the first clear explanation for the spectrum of human emotions. In the meantime, we can be both smugly pleased and profoundly disappointed that such emotions as joy, love, aggression, and fear are firmly rooted in the chemical soil of the brain. The fact may make us seem less human, but at the same time more wondrous in design. In addition, this discovery promises to yield some of the most effective treatments ever for mental disorders.

Rx for Schizophrenia

A cure for schizophrenia may reside in a combined regime of drugs, diet, and cleansing the blood of a chemical that may contribute to mental instability.

Diet

Schizophrenia is one of the most baffling of human states. Although psychiatrists disagree on its cause and treatment, there is mounting evidence that most, if not all, schizophrenia has a chemical basis. The biochemical theory most widely accepted today assumes that the symptoms of schizophrenia — disturbed thinking, perceptual distortions, paranoia, and withdrawal — result from having too much of the brain chemical dopamine and not enough of several other neurotransmitters: primarily acetylcholine (which the body manufactures from the choline in lecithin-rich foods) and the sleep-triggering hormone serotonin (which the body produces from the amino acid tryptophan, found in meats and dairy products). This theory has sparked several researchers to consider the role of diet in treating schizophrenia — as well as other kinds of mental illness. (See *Eating for Better Mental Health*, p. 17.) This is not a popular theory in psychiatric circles, but since several studies are in progress the theory is sure to make news, one way or another, during the 1980s.

Drugs

A more solid clue in solving the schizophrenia puzzle comes from the fact that researchers have detected abnormally large amounts of the naturally occurring brain proteins endorphins in the spinal fluid of acutely disturbed schizophrenics. Endorphins (for "endogenous morphine") are short strings of protein belonging to the peptide family of chemicals. They are structured like plant morphine molecules, and when extracted from the brain of animals and administered as a drug they display amazing painkilling properties.

Stanford University's Dr. Stanley Watson has found that the heroin antagonist naloxone, a chemical known to block the action of endorphins in the brain, has alleviated the auditory hallucinations in severely impaired schizophrenics. Patients besieged by imaginary voices are relived by comforting silence for up to two days on naloxone. What has confounded scientists is that a closely related brain protein, beta-endorphin, seems occasionally to cure schizophrenia. Psychiatrist Nathan Kline, director of the Rockland Research Institute in Orangeburg, New York, found that several chronic schizophrenics recovered and continued to improve more than ten months after their last beta-endorphin injection. One patient, a man who had been totally helpless for fifteen years, is now self-reliant. "There is very little doubt at the moment," says Dr. Kline, "that, for whatever reason, beta-endorphin is effective." The primary drawback to immediate treatment is its expense. A single injection of beta-endorphin costs $3000. Kline is certain, though, that the cost will soon decrease. If

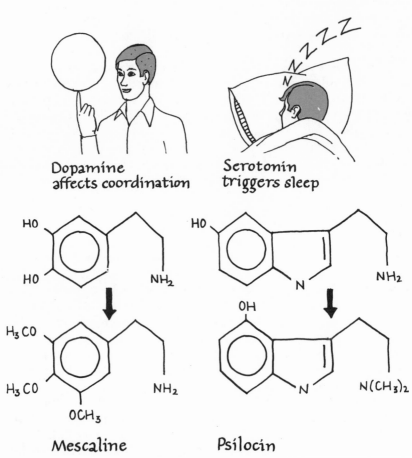

Dopamine
affects coordination

Serotonin
triggers sleep

Mescaline   Psilocin

Do Schizophrenics Produce Their Own Psychedelics?

Among their many roles, the brain chemicals dopamine and serotonin play roles in coordination and sleep, respectively. Interestingly, the chemical structures of these two neurotransmitters suspiciously resemble two potent hallucinogens, mescaline and psilocin (the active ingredient in psilocybin). In a chemist's language, mescaline and psilocin are methylated versions of dopamine and serotonin. Scientists are trying to determine whether the brains of schizophrenics manufacture hallucinogens, accounting for the voices, images, fears, and symptoms of withdrawal that characterize the disease. If this proves to be the case, new drugs could be developed to treat — and possibly prevent — schizophrenia.

similar studies confirm his observations, Kline asserts that clinical treatment of schizophrenia with beta-endorphin could be available by 1983.

Dialysis

Can your blood affect your mental health? Dr. Robert Cade, director of renal medicine at the University of Florida, has been putting diagnosed schizophrenics through six-hour blood-cleansing sessions as though they were being treated for kidney failure. He claims that more than half of the patients he has dialyzed since he began the treatment in 1972 "have either gotten well or improved enough to leave the hospital and go to work."

In 1978 Cade finally amassed evidence of why blood cleansing alleviates schizophrenic symptoms. The blood of his patients had contained an unusual brain protein called leucine endorphin in concentrations 10 to 100 times higher than normal. Each dialysis treatment removed more of the protein, and after the eighth week of treatment the leucine endorphin level had been reduced to a normal quantity. Cade's early success was considered suspect by most of his colleagues, but since the isolation of leucine endorphin several other researchers have tried dialysis — some with significant results. At the moment the evidence on dialysis is conflicting, and NIMH psychiatrists are investigating the technique. It may turn out that the causes of schizophrenia are varied: some patients might be helped by diet, others by drugs or dialysis. Or a combination of the three. One of mankind's oldest and most complex mental illnesses may be cured in our lifetime.

No More Cold Turkey

The brain's own proteins may provide the first testable theory — and the first innocuous cure — for drug addiction.

Enkephalins (based on the Greek for "in the head") are naturally occurring brain proteins. They differ from endorphins in that they are smaller protein chains, but like their chemical cousins they play a major role in the formation of emotions and perception of pain. It was in attempting to explain why morphine, a plant opiate, is such a powerful analgesic that researchers in 1975 first discovered enkephalins and endorphins. Thus, it's not surprising that the proteins may provide a cure for addiction.

Dr. Solomon Snyder of Johns Hopkins University has reason to believe that the dependence on an opiate like heroin (which structurally resembles the brain's own opiates) reduces the body's production of enkephalins. Therefore, greater quantities of heroin are needed as addiction continues, since the heroin must replace the missing enkephalins. The agony of withdrawal occurs because it takes the body time to resume its own production of enkephalins once heroin is stopped.

Several hospitals are testing Snyder's hypothesis. Some researchers radioactively tag heroin in order to chart its activity in the brain. Others are tracing the pathways of fluorescent-stained enkephalins. They hope to design a drug that temporarily compensates for the enkephalin deficit when an addict goes cold turkey, thus preventing the agony of withdrawal. Several new synthetic enkephalinlike drugs offer that possibility, but the trick is designing one that is itself nonaddictive. Computer drug design techniques hold out the promise that by the end of the 1980s such a nonaddicting drug will be available.

The Perfect Painkiller

A powerful, nonaddictive analgesic thousands of times more potent than morphine may be an early practical spin-off from modern brain research. Laboratories in Hungary, Switzerland, England, and the United States are competing to be first to market the superpainkiller — expected to be developed by 1985.

Chemically, the brain's natural opiates are dissimilar to morphine, which is an alkaloid — one of about twenty-five that together constitute opium. Enkephalins, on the other hand, are pentapeptides — molecules containing five amino acids (or simply a protein). In terms of geometrical structure, however, morphine and enkephalins both fit snugly into the same receptors in the brain. So when enkephalins were discovered in 1975, researchers immediately set out to develop their use as a perfect painkiller.

Of all the enkephalins they injected directly into the brains of hospitalized patients, they learned that only one, the C-fragment, acted as a powerful painkiller; it is in fact 100 times more potent than morphine. But a painkiller that must be injected into the brain is impractical. Enkephalins given intravenously provide only minor and very temporary pain relief because the brain's own protective enzymes quickly destroy foreign enkephalins as they try to pass from the blood stream into the brain.

As a result, researchers decided to design synthetic enkephalins

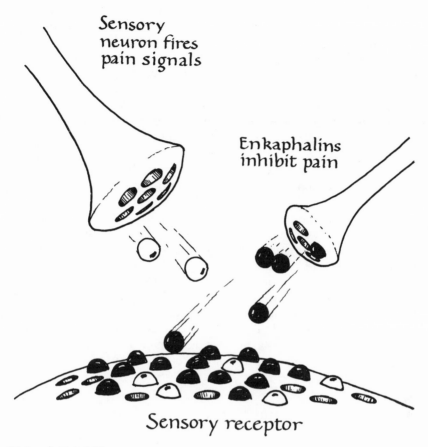

Sensory neuron fires pain signals

Enkaphalins inhibit pain

Sensory receptor

Nature's Painkiller

Tiny brain proteins called enkephalins rush to sensory receptors to block pain signals. The spinal fluid of patients wired with electrical stimulators that temporarily relieve pain contain increased amounts of enkephalins immediately after patients activate these stimulators. We may naturally produce varying amounts of enkephalins, accounting, in some cases, for variations in response to pain stimuli. A new generation of painkillers may operate by increasing the brain's enkephalin production.

to resist the attack of brain enzymes, and their efforts have begun to pay off. In 1976 Dr. Candace Pert of the Johns Hopkins University School of Medicine developed a synthetic enkephalin that offered profound, long-lasting relief when injected into rats. The following year Dr. Kastin at Tulane University discovered a synthetic enkephalin that relieved pain in rats for a period thirty times longer than natural enkephalins. Now drug companies have entered the field and are spending millions of dollars tinkering with amino-acid chains to find the perfect painkiller.

Scientists in Budapest have substituted two tiny amino acids into an enkephalin chain and come up with a chemical that, when injected into the human brain, has 1500 times the painkilling power of natural enkephalins. At Sandoz, Inc., in Switzerland, scientists have constructed an enkephalin analog that is 30,000 times more powerful than the brain's own version. What's most promising (and highly unusual) is that it retains its analgesic quality when taken orally, which had not been thought possible because peptides normally are digested before they can enter the blood stream and make their way to the brain. Unfortunately, Sandoz's present version of the superpainkiller is mildly addictive. Yet Swedish scientists feel that within a few years they will produce an addictive-free version of the drug. At present, opiates like morphine are unrivaled in dulling the severe pain that accompanies surgery, burns, and malignancies. In a few years' time however, these plant opiates, which can lead to addiction, may become obsolete.

Acupuncture and the Brain

Enkephalin research may provide the breakthrough in our understanding of how acupuncture relieves pain. The ancient Chinese claimed that acupuncture worked by balancing yin and yang energies; it now appears that strategically sticking the body with needles spurs the brain to release painkilling enkephalins.

Though most American scientists and physicians initially attributed acupuncture analgesia to a placebo effect, suggestibility, or hypnosis, they currently agree that pain relief by acupuncture can be genuine. In 1977 Dr. David Mayer at the University of Virginia School of Medicine experimented with acupuncture and enkephalin production. He subjected courageous volunteers to pain by administering electric shocks to their feet. First, he demonstrated that acupuncture significantly reduced their pain. Next, he injected his volunteers with naloxone, a chemical known to counter the effect of enkephalins, and again subjected them to electric shocks, under acupuncture therapy. Their adverse reactions — screams, jerks, and leg kicks — convinced him that naloxone had destroyed the analgesic benefits of acupuncutre. In Mayer's judgment, his experiment produced strong evidence that acupuncture minimizes pain by stimulating the brain to release enkephalins into the central nervous system. If this theory is accurate, it will constitute a major breakthrough — a biochemical explanation for a 5000-year-old medical art.

The Ultimate Trip

The perfect painkiller may also become a peerless pleasure pill, the "in" drug of the 1980s and 1990s. Development of the former will undoubtedly spawn an underground market for the latter.

If a super-synthetic enkephalin can alleviate pain, it should, theoretically, also induce blissful euphoria. Morphine, after all, plays both roles — and it and enkephalins act on the same nerves in the brain. The goal of brain researchers is not to produce a superpsychedelic, yet it already appears to be an offshoot of pain research. To test the pleasure potential of enkephalins, researchers at Wyeth Laboratories in Philadelphia implanted small tubes into the brains of rats. By pressing levers, the animals could freely tap solutions of enkephalins, morphine, and a neutral fluid. The rats opted for the enkephalins as often as for morphine, and seldom for the neutral shot. Enkephalins, the researchers concluded, induce pleasure similar to that of morphine.

The perfect painkiller ought not to be physiologically addictive, but as a potent mood elevator it could easily hook people psychologically. Drug-control authorities have fought against heroin-trafficking for over a hundred years; the black-marketing of the "peerless pleaser" could turn into the drug-control nightmare of the next century.

Fits of Pleasure

The great novelist Fyodor Dostoevsky experienced extraordinary euphoria prior to his epileptic seizures. Other epileptics have reported similar feelings. The pleasure-inducing ability of enkephalins may soon provide doctors with a biochemical explanation for epilepsy, and an original, highly effective treatment for the ailment.

In 1972 an epileptic submitted himself to electrical stimulation of the part of his brain called the amygdala. He was not cured, but he did experience opiumlike intoxication lasting for hours. This response mystified his doctors. Six years later neurologists discovered that the amygdala is rich in enkephalins, and they immediately posed the question: Do high concentrations of enkephalins produce epileptic seizures? In 1978 scientists at the University of California School of Medicine in San Francisco found the answer by injecting enkephalins into different areas of the brains of rats. In the rats' midbrain, enkephalins acted as painkillers; in the forebrain, they induced epileptic fits. It appears that epilepsy may result from tiny proteins that have wandered from their home base. Scientists suggest the possibility of developing a drug that would suppress enkephalin migration, or production in the forebrain, and this could become the preferred treatment for epilepsy.

Creative Drugs

Deep into a novel the writer is plagued by a mental block. A composer has written a brilliant first movement but can't shake clichés from the adagio. A million-dollar slogan eludes the ad executive. What they all have in common is a need for insight, which they may receive from the creative drugs of the 1990s.

Aldous Huxley believed that hallucinogenic drugs could inspire creativity and fresh ideas if only they didn't distort perception so strongly. Dr. Arnold Mandell, a psychiatrist at the University of San Diego, and Alexander Shulgin, a pharmacologist, are tinkering with hallucinogens to design a drug with precisely the properties Huxley dreamed of. Their findings are still tenuous, however, because testing new drugs on people must progress slowly. A psychiatrist at the University of Chile, Dr. Claudio Naranjo, has experimented with a few of Mandell's drugs on students and found that their thinking and emotions are heightened without perceptual distortion. One compound, developed from linking mescaline to a popular amphetamine, seems to produce neither euphoria nor speeding, but a sense of newness or novelty in a familiar situation. Another compound, made from manipulating a common antidepressant drug, not only relieves depression, but also creates feelings of high motivation. This experimental compound is being tested on mental patients and stands a good chance of becoming a commercial antidepressant.

Still, no pill can be expected to turn a dullard into a genius, or generate motivation where there's no underlying ambition. But if a person's creative instincts are blocked or have temporarily turned stale, he could receive a fresh boost from these psychotropic drugs. Dr. Mandell feels that for the most part performance-enhancing drugs will be illegally synthesized, tested behind closed doors, and sold on the black market. Perhaps by 1990. When will doctors be able to prescribe a creativity pill? "It will take decades," Mandell predicts. "There is no aegis in our society for introduction of performance or life-improving drugs. Under whose aegis, for instance, could we administer a creativity drug?"

12

Sleep Breakthroughs:
You'll Sleep to Be Healed

The Sleep-Death Connection

A link exists between the amount of time you sleep and how long you will live. There may even exist a Sudden Adult Death Syndrome that could be the primary cause of death among the elderly. One prominent sleep researcher, Stanford University's Dr. William Dement, believes that perhaps within a decade we'll be able to predict death — and thus delay it — by recording nocturnal sleep patterns.

The most healthful, soundest, and most restful sleep occurs in childhood and early adolescence. After about age sixteen the quality of sleep begins to deteriorate. Sleep is no longer always rejuvenating; it's often light, easily interrupted. And falling asleep is not as easy as it once was. In middle-to-late life several serious sleep problems surface: chronic insomnia, nocturnal myoclonus (hundreds of involuntary muscular leg kicks each night), alpha-delta syndrome (an unrestful mix of drowsiness and deep sleep), and sleep apnea (a form of strangulation). Why does the quality of sleep deteriorate with age? Is it a sign that the body, in general, is faltering?

Somnologists at the National Institute of Aging maintain that older people who sleep more than 10.5 hours or less than 4.5 hours may be on the threshold of death. They are experiencing "pathological sleep," an indicator that their bodies are in imminent danger. One recent study of persons over sixty-five stunned somnologists. They learned that more than 75 percent of the study group who slept just 1 hour more or less than the average 7.5 hours nightly were more likely to die. The link between sleep and death or disease is backed by several new findings:

• The onset of heart disease, stroke, cancer, and suicidal depression have all been connected with patterns of extremely long or very short nightly sleep.

• Older people who frequently rely on sleeping pills run a 50 percent higher risk of death. Hypnotic sleeping pills depress respiration. Elderly people naturally have less oxygen in their blood, so hypnotics increase their vulnerability to hypoxemia (deficient blood oxygenation) during sleep.

• Sleep apnea is a condition in which a person stops breathing and gasps for air with loud snores up to several hundred times a night. About 90,000 Americans, mostly the overweight and elderly, are believed to be afflicted with apnea, and Dr. Charles Pollak of the Montefiore Sleep-Wake Disorder Unit claims that a person suffering from apnea spends about 90 percent of his sleep time not breathing! "This can have profound effects on the cardiovascular system," he says. "We only see sleep apnea in patients under sixty, and I suspect that's because older people simply die from it."

NIA director Dr. Robert Butler suspects that psychological factors may also be instrumental in the sleep-death link: "There is a great desire to die in one's sleep" rather than while awake. Some researchers argue that nursing-home schedules may affect the time of death. Many operate on bizarre time schedules: patients get up at 4:00 A.M., have breakfast at 5:00, lunch at 10:00, supper at 5:00 P.M., and then are drugged to sleep. This dangerously disrupts biorhythms that are already on the decline as death approaches. Going to bed under these conditions can be fatal, and has probably killed thousands of people before their time.

Somnologists at the NIA are monitoring the sleep of people from ages forty to seventy, taking sophisticated measurements of cerebral blood flow, cardiac function, metabolism, and sleep's own stages. They hope to relate specific sleep abnormalities to the development of certain diseases and arrive at a "Prediction Profile." By the late 1980s this kind of profile may serve as an important tool in preventive medicine, a routine aspect of a physical examination, and a method of forecasting — and perhaps even forestalling — death.

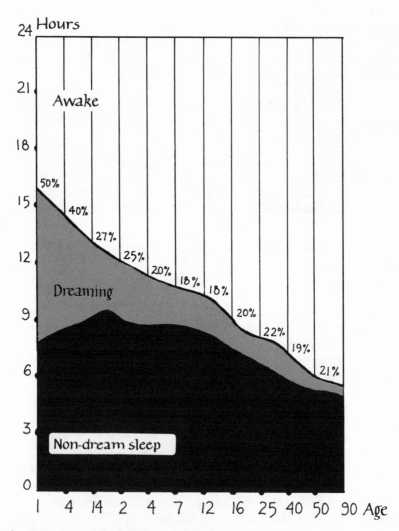

The Progression of Sleep over a Lifetime

Infants sleep almost sixteen hours a day, and dream (Rapid Eye Movement sleep) 50 percent of that time. Although the content of these dreams is, and probably always will remain, a mystery, an infant's REM sleep is thought to be the time he or she files into memory the abundance of the day's sensory stimuli — and perhaps copes with the traumas of life outside the womb. By old age the amount of REM sleep has fallen to a mere one hour (or about 21 percent of the night's total sleep time). On the other hand, the amount of non-dream (non-REM) sleep remains relatively more constant throughout a lifetime, progressing from roughly eight hours at birth to six hours in old age. Irregular sleep patterns eventually may be used to diagnose diseases and to predict — and perhaps forestall — death.

Sleep and Sex Problems

During 80 percent of rapid eye movement (REM) sleep, or dream sleep, men, regardless of age, usually have an erection. This experience is not connected with the sexual content of dreams, for when these men are awakened in sleep laboratories they relate prosaic dreams of playing golf, mountain climbing, and running from monsters.

Women, however, were thought not to experience arousal in sleep unless it was connected with a sexual dream. But in May 1978 researchers at the Memphis Mental Health Institute observed that during dream sleep, which occurs about four times a night, women experience increased blood in the genital tissues. As with men, the reason for this REM arousal remains a mystery. Researchers have serendipitously found, though, that men who don't have REM erections in sleep suffer from impotence when awake — regardless of whether the impotence has a psychological or physiological basis. The spectrum of women's sexual disorders is far broader than men's and the ailments harder to detect. Studies are in progress to learn if women with genital problems from infertility to vaginal and cervical cancer are subject to abnormal nocturnal REM arousal, and whether such patterns forecast the onset of these conditions.

By the mid 1980s sexologists hope to diagnose certain female sexual disorders while a woman sleeps. It could be the first of many clinical applications of the new diagnosis-in-sleep research.

Schizophrenic Sleep

Physical disease may not be the only illness to manifest itself in sleep. In the future such mental disorders as depression, mania, melancholia, and some forms of schizophrenia may be accurately diagnosed while a person is sleeping.

Judging by ongoing studies at the National Institute of Mental Health, patients suffering from affective disorders take longer to fall asleep, sleep for shorter periods of time, and move more rapidly and erratically into dream sleep than is considered normal. By examining electronically recorded sleep patterns, NIMH psychiatrists were able to diagnose correctly the mental states of about 80 percent of 115 patients in one study. The high diagnosis rate, the psychiatrists feel, lends further credence to the belief that many mental disorders are caused by faulty brain chemistry and that the sleep cycle is particularly sensitive to such chemical imbalances.

Research in the diagnosis of mental illness through sleep patterns is still in its infancy. Nonetheless, psychiatrists at George Washington University and at Mahelona Memorial Hospital in Kappa, Pauai, have been able to perform accurate diagnoses from sleep traces, and additional tests are scheduled. NIMH psychiatrists emphasize that no single brainwave pattern characterizes a specific mental disorder; rather, deviations among at least twelve sleep variables combine to suggest a diagnosis.

What Your Dreams Really Mean

Interpreting dreams made Freud famous and has helped psychoanalysis become the thriving profession it is today. However, future dream researchers may prove that your dreams contain no hidden symbolism or profound revelations at all. In fact, there may be really nothing mysterious about them.

Harvard psychiatrists Allan Hobson and Robert McCarley have already arrived at that revolutionary conclusion. They agree with Freud that dreams may be unique to your personality and experiences, but they disagree that the subconscious translates dreams into surreal, and supposedly meaningful, images. Dream images, they contend, amount to little more than the efforts of the logical brain trying to make sense of the body's electrical impulses it receives while you're sleeping.

From animal studies, Hobson and McCarley have concluded that dreams originate in the brain stem, an area that controls breathing, heartbeat, and other involuntary functions. These vital processes continue while you sleep, sending electrical impulses to those brain areas which control vision, memory, and emotions. When you're awake, your brain is too preoccupied to detect these sparks, but when you're asleep, your brain reads them. Often the signals don't correlate well (if at all) with real-world signals you're familiar with. So, commendably, your brain does its best to piece together fragments from your memory that nearly match the strange signals. That's why, for example, you may dream of flying, levitation, or being in two places at the same time.

The Harvard psychiatrists are convinced that the dream process can offer significant insights into how the brain works, but they caution that not too much substance should be attached to the meaning of dreams. A dream may not make sense, they assert, because it is more likely nonsense than profundity. If research in the 1980s supports their interpretation of dreams, their theory could strip dreaming of some of its fun — and a lot of its profit.

Dreaming to Remember

If you are to file away your memories of the day, it is essential that you dream. In short, no dreaming, no long-term memory.

Each of us has three to seven dreams — lasting from a few minutes up to an hour — during each eight-hour period of sleep. Since 1952 scientists have known that dreaming is always accompanied by rapid eye movements, REMs, but the function of REM sleep was not clear. In the 1960s French psychologists Vincent Block and Pierre Leconte showed that trained rats forgot how to navigate mazes after being deprived of REM sleep. Subsequently, Dr. Chester Pearlman, a Boston psychiatrist, observed that rats deprived of REM sleep after they had mastered an intricate system of avoiding electric shocks to get food starved to death when the tests were repeated. Lack of REM sleep, not fatigue, was responsible for the rats' forgetfulness.

Taking Pearlman's tests a step further, researchers at the University of Ottawa have learned that during REM sleep we integrate recently learned material into long-term memory. Working with a group of students enrolled in an intensive language course, the researchers discovered that students who pick up facts fastest tend to increase their amount of REM sleep, and slower learners record no increase. The discovery explains why students who stay up all night cramming for exams quickly forget the material they had absorbed. "You introduce a lot of facts that you really can't learn," says Pearlman. "The next day you won't be able to remember any of it, and you certainly will not be able to use any of it in the future — it is not part of you."

Why is dreaming necessary for remembering? No one is quite sure. Perhaps the more appropriate question is: Does the brain's process of filing information *produce* dreams? This suggests a ready, albeit incomplete, answer. As the brain files away data about various persons, places, and experiences you encounter each day, it also unconsciously glimpses some old fragments of material already on file. Suppose one night in the filing process your brain happens to scan your tenth birthday party, the face of a fraternity brother, or a NASA rocket launch you had watched on television. That night you might end up dreaming that you're on a launch pad, celebrating your tenth birthday, while former college friends toast you as rockets shoot out of the candles on your cake. But can that be the substance of dreams? Not entirely. Though current dream theory is moving in that general direction, there are nevertheless important questions for researchers of the 1980s to answer. Why, for example, did the brain choose certain old fragments and overlook others? Purely accidentally? Probably not.

During the 1980s researchers hope to arrive at a clearer picture of the relationship between dreaming and memory. In the meantime, if you are studying for a test, learning a language, or generally learning new information, it may be best not to stay up late cramming; instead, review the material at bedtime and then get a full eight hours sleep.

Dreaming to Reduce Stress

Dr. Pearlman and a colleague, Dr. Ramon Greenberg of Boston's Veterans' Administration Hospital, are persuaded that REM sleep aids us in coping with daily stress. Recording the sleep patterns of psychiatric patients, Pearlman and Greenberg discovered that a rise in REM sleep occurred after stressful discussions. In another experiment with nonpatients, they found that the need for REM sleep rose dramatically after the subjects had been shown distressing movies. As a result, the researchers concluded that the memory function and coping function of REM sleep are intimately linked and that sleep enables you to assimilate and adjust to traumatic experiences. Thus, if you try to escape a stressful situation by sleeping, you may actually be helping yourself adjust to stress. On the other hand, if you let the experience bother you enough to keep you awake, you may compound your problems.

Just how dream sleep allows you to cope with traumas should be more fully understood in the decade of the 1980s. But it is already clear that when Shakespeare wrote "To sleep: perchance to dream," he recognized only part of the story. Much more important for each of us is "To dream: perchance to cope."

13

Aging Breakthroughs:
You Won't Have to Grow Old

Aging as a Curable Disease

Eternal life will never be in our grasp, of course, yet an additional twenty to forty years is a real and not-so-distant possibility.

The reason for optimism comes from recent work with animals. Dr. Denham Harman of the University of Nebraska doubled the life span of mice by lacing their diets with such antioxidants as 2-MEA (2-mercaptoethylamine), vitamin E, and BHT (butylated hydroxytoluene, a preservative used in bread and canned foods). Then Harman discovered an unexpected payoff: offspring of these mice, though fed no antioxidants, also lived longer — apparently beneficiaries of their mothers' improved condition. We have not been given 2-MEA or BHT in such large doses, but the effects of vitamin E have been studied by Dr. Lester Packer of the University of California at Berkeley. Dr. Parker found that large amounts of vitamin E double the life span of human lung cells in test tubes.

Why do antioxidants prolong life? Proponents of the "oxidation theory" of aging believe that electrically active chemicals in the body, called free radicals, gradually bring about a sort of biological rusting of tissues and organs. Antioxidants act as sponges to sop up the rust-causing radicals and render them harmless.

Since there is no single accepted theory on aging, age-retardation research is branching along several paths. Some scientists view aging as a breakdown of the metabolic furnace. The principle is simple enough: the faster you force your metabolic furnace to burn up food, the sooner it gives out. For example, rats limited to 60 percent of their normal caloric intake (fasting one day in three) live a third to a half longer lives. Mice, deliberately underfed but given a nutritious diet, live to old age without the deteriorative signs of age. Until recently, limiting caloric intake — merely eating less — was believed to be beneficial only if started early in life, before puberty. But Dr. Charles Barrows of the National Institute on Aging has increased the life span of rats by as much as 33 percent by cutting their protein levels in half, starting at the age of sixteen months — the equivalent, according to Barrows, to the human age of forty-five.

A pill to retard aging, however, is at least twenty years in the future, and no one knows whether consuming large quantities of antioxidants has harmful side effects. But eating less, says Barrows, is something everyone can and should do. The secret is to eat a well-balanced, nutritious, low-calorie diet. It could prolong your life by as much as ten years.

Your "Death Hormone"

Your aging clock must first be located before it can be slowed down or set back. Biologists have narrowed their search to two sites in the body, both of which may be ticking away the years.

Wear and tear, once considered the primary causes of aging, have now been superseded by a biological clock. The ticking begins sometime between birth and puberty, but scientists are divided on whether the clock is hormonal in nature, residing in the brain, or whether it is in the DNA in every body cell.

In a clever series of experiments conducted thirty years ago, biologist Leonard Hayflick demonstrated that if the nucleus of an old cell was substituted for that in a young cell, the latter acquired the life expectancy of the former and soon died. More remarkable, when a young nucleus was transferred to an old cell, the cell gained a new lease on life. This experiment, often replicated, has convinced many gerontologists that the aging clock ticks in the DNA helix — with an alarm set to go off at roughly age seventy.

On the other hand, gerontologist Dr. W. Donner Denckla, formerly of the Roche Institute, is a leading proponent of another theory: that aging is triggered by a hormone that begins to be released by the pituitary gland at puberty. People do not really die of heart or kidney failure, liver malfunction or strokes, according to Denckla. These are merely the results of the failure of certain immune cells to deliver vital oxygen and nutrients to the organs that need them.

From his work with rats, Denckla has compiled evidence that the pituitary gland produces a chemical, yet to be isolated, that he calls DECO (decreasing oxygen consumption). Other scientists refer to it as the "death hormone." If the pituitary gland in an old rat is removed, the rodent stops aging; if it then receives the growth hormone thyroxine, a host of functions, from sturdier heartbeat to fresh fur growth, return to their youthful peaks. In contrast, animals with intact pituitaries that are given the growth hormone show no rejuvenation.

Naturally, we would not opt to have our pituitary removed, because the gland performs many life-supporting functions. However, once DECO has been isolated and synthesized — perhaps by 1983 — Denckla thinks that a chemical can be found either to prevent DECO's release or to render it inactive.

Biological Suicide

Dr. Hans Selye of the University of Montreal is following yet a different course in age retardation. Selye, a leading authority on the effects of stress, asserts that the deteriorative aspects of aging represent a perverse breakdown in the immunological system. According to Selye, your immune system, which throughout life fights vigorously against foreign invaders, suddenly turns against the body and literally commences to fight it to death. This genetically programed reversal may be prematurely triggered by the accumulated effect of years of stress, or set off by a major stressful incident such as the death of someone you love or the breakup of your marriage. Selye has discovered a group of elixirs, catatoxic compounds. When fed to rats, these chemicals apparently force the body to fight back against its own aging. "With catatoxic substances," says Selye, "we have made the first tentative steps in combating the disease to which we all succumb — aging."

Life's Elixir

Another possible reason for aging is that the brain slows down production of chemicals called catecholamines. In 1978 Dr. Caleb Finch at the University of Southern California demonstrated the chemical similarity of the brains of young and old animals — ex-

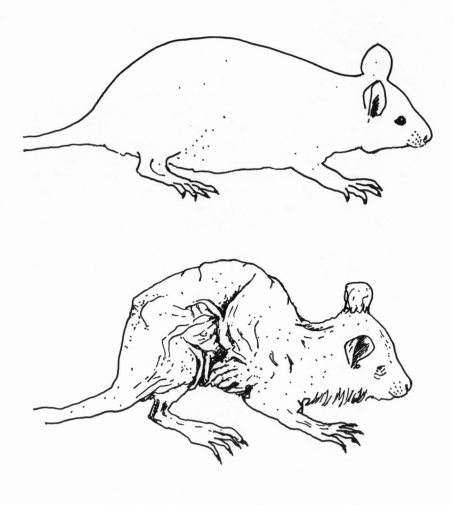

Two·month·old litter mates

The Chemistry of Youth

The bodily deterioration that characterizes aging may be rooted in biochemistry. These two rats from the same litter were fed a diet containing chemicals that accelerate the effects of time by producing the biochemical by-products of aging. The diet of the rat that looks its age (two months) also contained chemicals called catatoxic steroids, which counteracted the effects of the aging diet. The unprotected rat, after only four weeks on the aging diet, developed cataracts, a severely curved, weakened spine, and shriveled skin; by the end of the second month on the aging diet this rat could have been mistaken for its mate's grandfather. Catatoxic steroids, and other anti-aging chemicals, have not yet been tested on people.

cept for varying amounts of catecholamines, which existed in lower concentrations in the brains of older rats.

One catecholamine, dopamine, is of major importance in Parkinson's disease, a condition that strikes primarily older people. Finch speculates that aging may be "merely Parkinson's disease gone from bad to worse. Maybe if we all lived to be 150 we would develop Parkinson's disease." There are drugs available that increase the brain's production of catecholamines, but no one has yet tested them to determine if they have any effect on aging.

• • •

Whatever theory of aging, or combination of theories, proves correct, it is clear that in the not-too-distant future there will be drugs to prolong your life. Recently, two polls sampled the opinions of age-retardation scientists. Their optimistic assessment: by the year 2020 the human life span could be increased by as much as forty years.

Babies after Sixty

Your interest in sex may last well into old age, but it's common knowledge that your ability to procreate takes a precipitous dive. One day, however, couples in midlife may be able to have another child. And another. With no biological risk to mother or child.

Though rare, there are documented cases of men reproducing as late in life as ninety-four, and women as late as fifty-seven. But the average woman's reproductive capacity declines sharply between ages forty-five and fifty, as eggs are no longer released from her ovaries. Her vagina loses fat content, and although aging does not appear to wither the Fallopian tubes through which eggs once passed on their way to the uterus, the uterine walls quickly lose vital muscle protein. Although a man can usually reproduce to a later age than a woman, his testes shrink, he produces fewer sperm and fewer ejaculations, and his sperm are less mobile, less fertile, and often deformed.

What puts an end to procreation? Is sterility inevitable?

Intriguingly, the answer may reside not with a decrease in sex hormones from the gonads, as was considered to be the case, but with neurochemicals in the brain. (There have been a few anecdotal reports of injections of male sex hormones increasing older men's sexual drives. But there is stronger evidence that gonadal hormones are not solely responsible for reproduction. Steroid sex hormones administered to older women, for example, do not

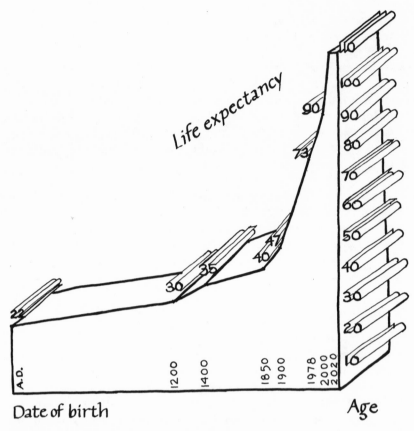

Life expectancy

Date of birth

Age

The Promise of an Additional Forty Years

Life expectancy at birth has been rising steadily throughout recorded history. (The frightfully low average for many centuries was largely due to high infant mortality.) A sharp increase in life expectancy began about 100 years ago, and this climb is expected to continue, even more steeply, as a result of anticipated advances in age-retardation research. A realistic estimate is that by the year 2020 the average life expectancy at birth may be 110 years of age.

lengthen their reproductive years.) Dr. Gail Riegle of Michigan State University has proved that a decrease in the nerve transmitter norepinephrine switches off the reproductive cycle in rats. Female rats chemically induced to produce more norepinephrine conceive in old age and bear normal offspring. Effete male rats subjected to the same treatment produce as much testosterone as they did in their prime. So evidently the onus for reproductive aging is not on the gonads, but on the central nervous system.

Riegle theorizes that human conception could be extended well beyond the fifty-year cut-off point for women, and even further for men. Chemicals that activate the brain's crucial neurotransmitters already exist but have yet to be tested in extending reproduction. If they work, and produce no dangerous side effects, a couple well into middle age would have to weigh their desire for more children against possible disadvantages — to the couple and the children — of their becoming parents late in life. But, then, if an age-retardation pill is available as well, fifty could be the prime of life.

Thinking Clearly at 120

The purpose of age-retardation research is to add useful, productive years to your life. No one wants to live to 120 if senility sets in at ninety. Hand in hand with the goal to prolong life is the quest to keep you mentally sharp in old age.

In old age the arteries in the head as well as the heart are likely to become atherosclerotic. As a result, the brain, deprived of adequate blood, becomes starved for oxygen, begins to falter and forget.

In tests at Emory University in Atlanta, Dr. C. Doyle Haynes has shown that the I.Q. and personality of people over age fifty-seven are significantly improved after their carotid arteries are scoured by an operation known as endarterectomy. This flushing procedure has been used to prevent strokes, but it may constitute a means to reverse the onset of senility.

Carotid artery occulsion is remarkably common. Probably 10 percent of the population under age fifty suffer from it, and 40 percent of those over fifty have badly clogged arteries. Thus, for many people, impairment of brain function starts in middle age.

Haynes's patients — the oldest was eighty — were aware of their increased mental acuity. Tests proved that their verbal comprehension, perception, and analytic-reasoning skills improved, and the oldest patients displayed a "general reduction of suspicion, distrust, and disorientation" that had marked their previous behavior.

It is a hopeful sign, says Haynes, that senility is due not to gradual deterioration of brain cells (in fact, they appear to be the hardiest, longest-living cells in your body), but mainly to a clogging of the arteries, which cuts off oxygen and nutrients to the brain.

Endarterectomies are already enabling people to live fuller lives, and the operation is bound to become more popular.

The Social, Political, and Religious Impact of Anti-Aging Pills

The forecasts below are a composite of those made by thirty-one graduate students in future studies at the University of Houston. After studying reports on age-retardation research, the students constructed scenarios depicting the effects that a drastic extension of life might have on society.

	One Year after the introduction of the anti-aging pill	Ten Years after the introduction of the anti-aging pill
Personality	There is an extremely wide range of reactions to the anti-aging pill. Most people are happy and some are euphoric, but a sizable minority are confused and disoriented, especially those with strongly held religious beliefs. Physiological side effects are rumored, creating yet greater indecisiveness.	With virtually everyone taking the anti-aging pill by now, adults in this society resemble adolescents in the pre-pill days, in that they are mercurial, introverted, uneasy, and casting about for purposes and alliances. Their sights have been lifted to a much more distant horizon, but they are unsure how to fill up the great expanse before them. They are generally less aggressive than before, but some of the young resent the old getting younger. Suicide becomes more common than ever before, reaching a peak that it will never again attain.
Family Life	Differing opinions about the safety or effectiveness of the pill bring an increase in tension within families. Divorce rates rise as couples shun spending eternity together, but so do birth rates, as parents who anticipate limits on new births decide to have children now.	There is no doubt that the traditional family structure is breaking down. The divorce rate ascends, marriage becomes uncommon, and much more amorphous groupings appear. Since the number of children per family is prescribed by policy (but still not by law), the dipping number of children results in great attention and good will for each youngster.
Education	Educators are demoralized as they recognize that their traditional clientele of children and adolescents cannot continue.	The educational system finds renewed purpose, because it must bear much of the burden of adjustment from mortal to immortal society. Emphasis is shifting from children to adults and from degree-granting programs to courses relating to careers and leisure experiences.
Leisure	Dangerous sports such as auto racing and boxing begin to lose participants. Increased sales of games and other diversions do not yet materialize, due to the disorientation of the public.	Contact sports die out, to be replaced by thrilling but not dangerous activities. Loosely organized tournaments are held for popular games, much like the pre-pill Frisbee tournaments. Travel greatly increases.

Employment and the Economy	The economy threatens to destabilize. Businesses work frantically to analyze what prolonged lives will mean to their markets and products. Some employees desert their positions and others hold tenaciously onto their jobs as the more far-sighted and callous of businesses try to prune away the deadwood. There is little hiring going on, and unemployment rises to 8%.	The economy is slowing down. Production is increasingly automated as labor becomes difficult to handle. Although unemployment is high, so is absenteeism. Initiative and morale of employees is slight. Job mobility is low. Pension plans have received permission to disband.
National Government	It is immediately obvious to all that the government will have to assume a larger role in order to handle the discontinuities caused by the anti-aging pill. The government has been quick to take over the distribution of the pill (but not the production) and to curtail any efforts by officials to tenure themselves. Major problems have been identified and the debates have begun already: whether or not people such as habitual criminals or the insane, or even house pets, should be given the pill; how birth limitations are to be imposed; how employment and retirement questions are to be determined.	Public confidence in the government remains high. The major dilemma occurs in enforcing the hard decisions about who will *not* get the pill. Decisions about legally binding birth limitations continue to be postponed, although the problem receives constant scrutiny. The government has legislated away all retirement plans and in some respects is beginning to take responsibility for the job market.
International Affairs	There is rapid worldwide diffusion of the pill, except in some Communist countries, where they are initially resisted. The confusion found in the American public is amplified abroad, especially in nations where traditional religions are strong. Outbreaks occur against governments slow to facilitate the distribution of the pill.	Belligerency between nations steadily decreases. Not only does no one wish to die for his country, but the realization grows that the people here now will be together for eternity. The problem of how global wealth will be distributed receives greater attention as productivity falls off faster in less-developed countries, where the labor force is becoming intractable. Insurrections occur in a few areas where pill distribution is incomplete, or where birth limitations are resisted.
Spiritual Matters	Traditional religions mount a campaign against the pill, although some Protestant groups try to accommodate themselves to it. The media carry acrimonious debates over the pill, the meaning of life, and the hereafter. After a short-lived increase in church attendance, a steady decline ensues.	Organized religions are largely disgraced and disbanded. Cults devoted to the self or the environment gain members.

	Twenty Years after the introduction of the anti-aging pill	Fifty Years after the introduction of the anti-aging pill
Personality	Low levels of discontent and distress remain, but for the most part tensions have eased. Religious and medical reservations about the pill have totally disappeared. Individuals are characterized by their thoughtfulness and caution. There is little competition and risk-taking.	While people remain safety-conscious and cautious, they are less introspective than before. They are generally acquiescent, content, and somewhat curious.
Family Life	The end of the family is in sight, since less than 25% of the population is married. Increasing in popularity are fluid groupings of 12 to 30 adults. The very few children around are indulged and treasured.	The family has officially disappeared. Condominium life is the most common living arrangement, where relations are intense, but short-lived and nonintrusive.
Education	Continuing education is by far the commonest mode, with courses open to all. There are courses for new jobs, for leisure activities, for the inculcation of wisdom. New information and knowledge is being generated at an even faster pace than ever before, since the life of a scholar is attractive to many and since computers can now do most of the rote work of any scholarly quest.	Education is not only funded but also directly administered by the federal government. Its services continue as before, with standards of teaching and scholarship reaching new heights. Automation has made few inroads in higher education. Polls reveal it to be the most respected institution.
Leisure	As thrill-seeking becomes less common, the use of recreational drugs reaches new heights. Taboos against any form of physical intimacy have disappeared. Having an abundance of free time, people turn to travel, games, the arts, and so on in even greater numbers. There is an enormous strain on public facilities.	The distinctions between leisure and education, and between leisure and work, are rapidly disappearing. Most people consider all these activities to be pleasurable and instructive.
Employment and the Economy	GNP is now rising at less than 1% annually. Production has become so automated that the need for labor is steeply decreased. Employment has been taken over and coordinated by the government. While all must work, there is so little work to be parceled out that individuals spend only 10 hours a week for 8 months at a job, then have 4 months off. While the fit between jobs and individual interests cannot be perfect, most are satisfied with the system for the varied experiences it provides them.	Although long heralded, it is not until now that automation has become so sophisticated that it extends beyond production and into management. The economy, whose ups and downs are minimal, is largely operated by computers. The labor force does no rote work, but generates new knowledge leading to improved performance.

National Government	The paternalistic government still enjoys wide popular support. The decision that anti-aging pills would contain birth control medication is being successfully enforced. The administration of employment is now the government's major obligation following the dismemberment of the Department of Defense. The government has formed the first 100-year economic plan, which is premised on a steady-state economy.	With the development of computer systems that can administer government agencies, most of the government's responsibilities have become routine. One area still receiving human attention is the development of recreational facilities. People look nostalgically upon the government, whose presence they perceive to be fading.
International Affairs	Increased cooperation, increased travel, and greater sharing of wealth all lead toward a lessening of distinctions between nations. New supranational governmental entities are beginning to form. Global planning is not yet in place, but is expected soon.	A well-managed global community is now in existence. Feelings of brotherhood run high.
Spiritual Matters	There is an extraordinary rise in attentiveness to the physical environment as awareness increases that humans are their own posterity, and that the earth is their habitat forever. Devotion to the environment assumes near-religious proportions.	The environment continues to be revered, but attention is turning again to the entire universe, whose origins and evolution are finally comprehended.

14

Behavior Breakthroughs:
How You'll Live, Work, and Love

Rearing Your Baby

Psychologists focused their attention on adolescents in the 1960s, and on midlife adults in the 1970s. In the 1980s they'll shift their focus once again, this time to study babies. The new insights into a baby's knowledge and how it learns are sure to shed light on numerous problems that confront us in adolescence and adulthood, teaching us to cope with them in much more efficient ways.

The world of the newborn was once thought to be filled by a pastiche of sounds, smells, and shadows. Infants scanned their environment indiscriminately, learning by trial and error. And during the formative weeks parents were virtually helpless in orchestrating the symphony of stimuli a baby perceived. Well, such notions couldn't be further from the truth. New studies are revealing that an infant still wet from the womb is far from a "blank slate."

Vision

As soon as a baby opens his eyes, he is attracted to adult faces, particularly eyes, which are now believed to play a crucial role in bonding an infant to his mother. To discover which features of the human face a baby prefers, Robert Frantz of Western Reserve University showed infants three flat figures the size and shape of a head. The first illustration was a human face painted pink and black, the second had scrambled facial features, and the third was a solid black patch. All the four-day-old babies tested were drawn most to the first drawing and least to the black patch. And when when they were given the additional choice of a real face, the babies immediately preferred it; tracking cameras revealed that the babies were mesmerized by eyes. Before too long researchers hope to know whether eye movement itself fascinates an infant, or whether from birth a baby actually perceives mood and emotion, which are so readily reflected by our eyes.

Hearing

Immediately after birth an infant recognizes the human voice and prefers it to any other sound, including music. Acoustic studies show that babies respond better to high frequencies than low ones. It is interesting that when we talk to babies, we automatically pitch our voice higher.

Coordination

A newborn can't walk, sit upright, or hold up his head. Yet, even though he lacks major muscle coordination, he possesses conceptual coordination to a surprising degree. At the University of Edinburgh, Thomas Bower created the optical illusion of an object in front of newborns. Strapped upright in supportive chairs, the babies reached for what they thought was an object, groping around the illusion to the point of great frustration. To Bower, these reactions offer strong evidence that coordination between eyes and hands is present at birth, and that newborns expect to be able to touch objects they see. Recent research has also shown that babies move in precise cadence to human speech, even though their movements are so subtle that they must be carefully observed.

Taste

An infant is born with a sweet tooth and an evident dislike for tastes salty and sour. Lewis Lipsitt of Brown University has demonstrated taste preference by offering liquids of varying sweetness to two-day-old babies. Without exception, every baby sucked longest and hardest on the sweetest solution, and their heartbeats raced. Other studies have also shown that newborns refuse to suck fluids even slightly salty or sour. Is it because a baby's body needs glucose, which it can make from sugar? Or is there a more fundamental genetic reason? Sweet-tasting leaves and berries are the safest jungle vegetation to eat; bitter plants are usually poisonous. This fact of life, so vital for primitive man, may be coded in our genes.

The business of baby-watching is a new scientific sport, and the facts being uncovered are beginning to have considerable impact on many of our cherished theories of social development. New emphasis is being placed on the importance of not only the early days after birth, but also the first hours of life. Some psychologists are already surrounding newborn infants with continuous music and color-discrimination projections, and are engaging infants in feats that require great coordination. How much — and how fast — can these new minds learn? How will I.Q. and personality be influenced by the selective presentation to infants of rich, nurturing stimuli? The answers will come too late to benefit directly anyone who reads these words, but perhaps in time to benefit our children.

Choosing a Career of Crime

Some kids steal, bully their friends, and shun the love showered on them. Eventually, they grow up to rob, rape, and kill. All attempts to rehabilitate them fail, and they become career criminals. Until recently, psychologists believed certain forms of mistreatment and poverty bred these kid-to-adult criminals, and that they were psychotics. But according to a bold new theory of the criminal mind, some kids just choose to be criminals, the way others opt to be lawyers, teachers, or musicians; otherwise, they're normal. Action based on this theory could prevent many of these children from choosing a life of crime, and at the same time revolutionize our penal system and result in the dismantling of most of our current rehabilitation programs.

In 1960 psychiatrist Dr. Samuel Yochelson began an intensive study of 252 hard-core male criminals at St. Elizabeth's, a hospital for the mentally ill in Washington, D.C. In searching for a mental and psychological basis for criminal behavior, Yochelson used conventional psychoanalytic techniques on his subjects, and ran batteries of blood, hormone, and chromosome tests. By 1965, however, he had made no progress in defining this basis and was forced to conclude that "psychiatric concepts and techniques don't work with criminals, because most diagnoses of mental illness result from the criminal's fabrications."

Yochelson then adopted a clever approach that he called the "stream of thinking." He instructed each criminal to "forget the past, concentrate on the here and now and report on your thoughts every day." Forced to talk about the present, the criminals found it more difficult to fabricate, and Yochelson was able to gain fresh insight into the criminal mind. Among his startling findings:

• The career criminal deliberately chooses a life of crime, even if it means traveling to other neighborhoods to find thrills and others of his kind to impress.

• From childhood he has obsessively craved power and the use of that power to intimidate.

• For the career criminal, lying comes as naturally as breathing. If he's going to a movie, he'll say it is *Superman* even if he plans to see *Star Wars*.

• The hard-core criminal derives thrills from just contemplating crimes he couldn't possibly commit. For instance, he may spend hours peering into store windows, planning ways to steal the merchandise.

• Confirmed criminals do not behave impulsively, as do psychotics; they weigh every risk, and act only when they feel that they can get away with their crime.

• Behind the criminal's macho façade hides a weak, cowardly individual. As a child he harbored abnormally strong fears of the dark, the doctor, thunder and lightning, and ghosts. He overcame these anxieties because of his far greater fear of being ridiculed by others.

Yochelson and Dr. Stanton Samenow, who joined the project in 1970, also studied more than 100 hard-core criminals who had been judged "not guilty by reason of insanity" and concluded that not a single diagnosis held up under scrutiny. They analyzed existing rehabilitation programs and devised and tried new ones, only to conclude that crime is so intrinsic to the hard-core criminal's personality that very few can be measurably helped.

Though their seventeen-year, federally funded study has understandably stirred heated controversy, many prison psychologists have greeted the report with overwhelming praise. Samenow feels that one significant method for reducing crime in society is by the early identification of criminal personalities. Perhaps within a decade, doctors and parents could be trained to spot potential criminal behavior in children, and, possibly, hints of antisocial behavior in infants. No one has yet catalogued the many factors that must converge in a child's mind to forge a criminal personality, much less proved whether the new theory is correct. But if a child who displays abnormal fears, enjoys intimidating his playmates, and rejects all kindness could be taught to overcome this behavior and increase his self-respect, then we as a society would surely stand to gain. In the decades ahead, the Yochelson-Samenow theory may lead to a major restructuring of our penal system and our means of rehabilitating criminals.

Sex Scents

Can your body scents sexually arouse others? There is growing evidence that they can. Chemists are close to isolating human fragrances that may influence your sex drives. And once synthesized, you can be sure that manufacturers will be adding these fragrances to everything from perfume to golf balls.

Odors from chemicals called pheromones are already known to affect the sexual behavior of insects. Male moths confronted with a rag doused with bombykol — an aphrodisiaclike pheromone secreted by female silk moths — exhibit their instinctive copulatory gyrations *with the rag*. Though the pheromone messages are primitive, they are irresistible. They have been successfully used in pest-control programs to lure swarms of unsuspecting males into fields where they devote their amorous attentions to leaves and twigs.

In laboratory experiments the sexual cycles of female rats, rabbits, dogs, and monkeys have also been manipulated through male urine scents from each species. Evidence is growing that men and women possess special sexual scents as well, and that some of us secrete more than others.

French scientist J. Le Magnen first demonstrated in 1952 that women were sensitive to the substance exaltolide, a musky fragrance secreted predominantly in men's urine and included today in several perfumes. More recent studies have confirmed that exaltolide does indeed sexually affect females. For instance, women who have had their ovaries removed lose their ability to detect exaltolide but regain it once they are treated with hormones. Interestingly enough, a woman's sensitivity to exaltolide peaks during ovulation — an evolutionary implication that exaltolide may have served as a primeval cue for survival of the human race.

A Feminine Fragrance

A female "sex" odor, however, has been harder to find. Attempting to test the old wives' tale that women who live together experience synchronized menstrual cycles, psychologist Martha McClintock studied 135 dormitory residents at Wellesley College in 1971. She learned that menstrual cycles of roommates and close friends began to coincide as the school year progressed. Her data hinted that the synchronizing factor was perspiration odor. Six years later a California study backed her suspicion.

In one experiment cotton pads were placed under the arms of women. These pads were rubbed daily against the upper lips of women in a second group, and gradually their periods became synchronous with those of the first group. Menstrual synchrony may be based on odiferous messages in female sweat, but is there a female scent that affects males?

Several laboratories are experimenting with certain natural chemicals, volatile fatty acids called copulins, that are found to varying degrees in the vaginal fluids of women. Copulins were discovered in 1974 by Michael Russell of the Emory University School of Medicine in Atlanta when he chemically analyzed tampons worn during menstruation. Russell reported that nearly all the women (97.5 percent) showed traces of copulins.

But are copulins aphrodisiacs? Research being done by Naomi Morris of the University of Chicago Medical School and Richard Udry of the University of North Carolina suggests that they may be. In the past, Morris and Udry have shown that human sexual intercourse peaks during the ovulation phase of the menstrual cycle, and that production of copulins also peaks at this time. In their present work, the two researchers had married women dab four different perfumes (one containing copulins) between their breasts at bedtime. The next morning the husbands and wives were asked to fill out individual questionnaires about their sexual feelings and activities of the previous night. Did copulins, in fact, increase the frequency of intercourse? Most men seemed unaffected, though a few claimed to be inspired to new sexual heights.

So far, no definite link has been established between sex scents and sexual behavior, but several more studies are underway. All chemical substances currently being investigated are secreted through the urine or by the apocrine glands in the underarm and genital areas. If pheromones are a remnant of our evolutionary past, it could be that our society's obsession with cleanliness and deodorants is overpowering the few remaining sex-signaling molecules we have.

Some scientists are confident that they will be able to isolate specific sex scents in the near future. Such bodily secretions, however, may turn out to be too insignificant to influence sexual behavior in most people. But once synthesized, various secretive concentrations could be tried to determine arousal levels for men and women. A bottle kept on the night table could save a marriage. Two whiffs of a prescribed scent may cure impotence, frigidity, and other sexual dysfunctions, as well. On the other hand, the potential abuse of such substances is mind-boggling. Sex scents could easily replace pot, poppers, and coke as the "in" drugs of the 1980s. And a line of sex-scented consumer products could keep us all so sexually aroused that we would do very little in the way of work.

Factory Fever

A woman on an assembly line packing frozen vegetables smells a strange odor. Minutes later she develops a headache and burning eyes. Co-workers suddenly experience similar symptoms, and the production line grinds to a halt. Within an hour women all over the plant fall ill — and the factory is forced to close. Investigators are brought in to search for some noxious chemical, toxic gas, or infectious bacteria. They find none. The women are diagnosed as suffering from "mass psychogenic illness" — a disease caused by psychological rather than physical factors.

The malady, discovered only recently by psychologists at the National Institute of Occupational Safety and Health, primarily strikes women factory workers. It spreads by contagion like a yawn and often produces such severe nausea, dizziness, and headaches that victims must be hospitalized. Since 1976, NIOSH psychologists have, with increasing frequency, documented cases of mass psychogenic illness. Recently, at a garment-manufacturing plant in Atlanta, Georgia, half of the 330 women employees were striken within a week. All shared nearly identical symptoms, and 18 had to be hospitalized. An exhaustive epidemiological investigation by city and state health officials and specialists from the Center for Disease Control failed to uncover a single physical clue.

It is hard to determine whether cases of mass psychogenic illness might have gone undiagnosed in the past, but there is growing evidence to indicate that it's a disease peculiar to modern-day living — and the incidence of it is definitely on the rise.

What causes a psychological epidemic? Why are victims almost always women? How do the symptoms spread so fast?

NIOSH psychologists are struggling to answer these questions, and hope that they will soon be able to diagnose, treat, and possibly prevent the disease — perhaps by 1984. So far, their research has pinpointed the fact that assembly-line workers who can't easily communicate with one another because of noisy machinery, staggered breaks, or short lunch periods are the most likely victims. Mass boredom caused by tedious work appears to predispose people to mass psychogenic illness. Some psychologists speculate that the disease may be especially common among working women because many of them have been forced by financial necessity to work when they would prefer the traditional woman's role in the home.

NIOSH psychologists think they understand how mass psychogenic illness spreads so quickly. A number of workers first experience mild, independent symptoms caused simply by frustration or fatigue. They reveal these complaints, however, only after seeing a co-worker — "the initiator" — fall ill. The initiator happens to be so near the point of physical or emotional collapse that any strange smell, peculiar noise, or suspicious puff of smoke pushes her over the brink.

NIOSH psychologists have begun to develop a battery of tests to identify workers particularly prone to mass psychogenic illness. The tests, the first research protocol for handling a psychological epidemic, may be adopted by the military, which has often reported group psychomatic ailments. One fear psychologists have is that companies may misuse these tests to screen out "susceptible" workers. In that case, a person rejected for a factory job may be able to sue the company for psychological discrimination.

Hyperactive Children

Scientists at the National Institute of Mental Health believe they are close to a breakthrough in understanding the cause of hyperactivity in children. In a few years they may even have designed a physical index for distinguishing hyperactive children from normal children. This would represent a major advance in diagnosing hyperactivity, and may save many normal children suspected of being hyperactive the trauma of drug therapy.

About 20 percent of schoolchildren are considered hyperactive, and of this group boys outnumber girls six to one. Many of these children are heavily drugged when they attend school, because amphetamines have been clearly demonstrated to relieve hyperactivity's major symptoms of inattentiveness and the inability to sit still in class. No one has figured out why "uppers" calm down hyperactive children. Nor do they know the causes of hyperactivity, though an endless string of possible causes includes refined sugar, fluorescent lights, tight underwear, food additives, hypoglycemia, and undiscovered organic illnessess.

Diet

The food-additive theory gained popularity in 1973 when allergist Dr. B. F. Feingold at the Kaiser-Permanente Medical Center in San Francisco claimed that 50 percent of the hyperactive children he treated recovered when he eliminated from their diet foods containing synthetic colors, synthetic flavors, and salicylates. A major study at the University of Wisconsin in 1977 failed to confirm Feingold's claim, but doctors are still uncertain which research is correct. Many physicians and parents swear by the Feingold diet.

Diagnosis

Neither electroencephalograms nor neurological examinations help to diagnose hyperactivity. Many physicians have resorted to the "paradoxical response" of amphetamines as a diagnostic tool: if a child believed to be hyperactive is calmed by large doses of amphetamines, then he is hyperactive. The accuracy of the circular logic has been hard to test because it would involve giving potentially dangerous drugs to hundreds of normal children who would have to serve as a control group. Scientists at the NIMH recently broke through this ethical barrier by studying boys aged six to twelve whose parents were in the medical profession and were fully informed of the nature of the study. Surprisingly, the normal children responded to a single dose of amphetamines the same way as the hyperactive children — both groups were affected by decreased motor activity and performed better on cognitive tests.

This seems to rule out one of the most routinely used diagnostic tests for hyperactivity, but another group at the NIMH believes there may be biological differences between hyperactive and normal children that would offer a means of diagnosis. Hyperactive children seem to have more of what doctors call minor physical anomalies — such as asymmetric or malformed ears, a curved fifth finger, a wide gap between the second and third toe, and abnormal reflexes. Fathers of hyperactive children also appear to have an unusually high number of these minor physical anomalies; some are so minor that they can go unnoticed by both parents and those born with the defects. Researchers suspect that these anomalies occur in the fetus early in pregnancy — perhaps during the first few weeks — and that whatever causes them may also lead to minor defects in the development of the central nervous system that are later manifested as hyperactivity.

More tests are necessary before researchers can design an index of physical traits that could be helpful in diagnosing hyperactivity. One danger, however, in devising such an index is that babies born with a large number of so-called hyperactive traits — who may otherwise be perfectly normal — could be diagnosed as hyperactive and treated as though they were, turning the diagnosis into a self-fulfilling prophecy. Over the next decade, NIMH scientists hope to test their theory that the roots of hyperactivity stem from early pregnancy problems. Once those problems can be identified, it may be possible for a mother to take preventive measures in the early weeks of pregnancy to decrease her child's chances of becoming hyperactive later in life.

15

Biometeorology Breakthroughs:
How Weather Affects Your Health

Weather-Related Diseases

How do humidity and barometric pressure combine to aggravate arthritis? What is weather's contribution to the spread of an epidemic? Why do seasonal changes influence ulcers and suicide rates?

Biometerology is the science that studies interactions between the two most complex systems on earth: man and weather. And although scientists have only recently developed the tools to study meteorotropic, or weather-related, diseases, the idea that a link exists between health and weather dates back to Hippocrates, who in 400 B.C. recorded physical and psychological reactions to hot and cold winds. Unfortunately, the next 2400 years are filled with myth, folklore, and home remedies for colds, creaking joints, and plagues that may have killed more people than they cured.

Arthritis

One weather-related ailment under intensive investigation is arthritis. To study the link between arthritis and weather, Dr. J. L. Hollander of the University of Pennsylvania placed arthritic patients in climate-controlled chambers. According to folklore, increased humidity aggravates this condition. Yet Hollander learned that increasing the humidity in the chamber was not sufficient to trigger arthritic pain and swollen joints; at the same time, barometric pressure had to fall. But how do atmospheric changes penetrate the body? Hollander suspects that the membranes in the joints act like an aneroid barometer. When barometric pressure is high, the membranes contract (like the plates in a barometer); as barometric pressure falls, the membranes expand, exerting a painful force on the bursae, pouchlike cavities that contain fluid to reduce friction between joints. If Hollander is right, the body mechanics underlying arthritis should help researchers develop more effective drugs to combat the ailment. In the meantime, when an arthritic person listens to a weather forecast he should pay more attention to barometric pressure than to the humidity predictions.

Colds

Is the common cold meteorotropic? Despite undeniable evidence that flu and sore throats peak in the winter months, scientists at the National Oceanic and Atmospheric Administration are discovering that the cold is not caused by weather—at least, not directly. Colds are nonexistent in polar regions and occur there only when passed on by visitors. Common cold viruses, in fact, can't survive extreme temperatures. Like us, viruses prefer temperate weather. NOAA scientists have found that in moderate latitudes cold viruses exist in about equal numbers during summer and winter. Apparently the incidence of colds peaks in winter because we are confined indoors, breathing "used" stale air, in which concentrations of viruses (as well as allergens and spores) can accumulate. There is mounting evidence that such stale air can be freshened, and thus cleansed of bacteria and viruses, with generators that produce charged particles called air ions. (See *Ions for Your Health*, p. 161.)

Cancer

Recently uncovered connections between events on the sun and the earth's weather are giving biometeorologists new insight into certain diseases. One such disease is skin cancer. There is nothing mysterious in the fact that excessive exposure to sun causes skin cancer. Scientists have known for years that workers in grape vineyards develop cancer on the back of the neck and hands, and never on the face, which is shielded in shadow. But the cancer-weather link can be deviously subtle. Scientists at the University

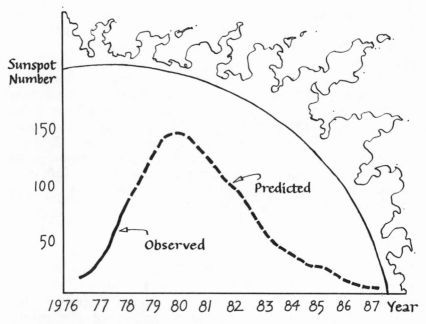

Beware of the Sun in 1980

Sunspot activity rises and falls in eleven-year cycles. The current cycle is expected to reach its maximum level of activity in 1980. Scientists have found evidence that three years after a sunspot maximum the incidence of skin cancer increases. The reason may be that an abundance of cosmic rays bombard the earth during periods of intense sunspot activity, depleting the ozone layer, which normally serves as a shield against the sun's carcinogenic ultraviolet light.

of Connecticut Medical School found that the incidence of skin cancer rises dramatically with the eleven-year sunspot cycle. They suspect the reason is bound up with the phenomenon of cosmic rays bombarding the earth during solar storms and depleting the ozone layer that normally shields the earth from most of the sun's carcinogenic ultraviolet light. Checking meteorological records and reported occurrences of skin cancer over many years, the University of Connecticut scientists have recorded a sharp rise in skin cancer almost exactly three years after a period of maximum sunspot activity. Soon they'll be able to test their theory. Sunspot activity will again reach a maximum in 1980. If the scientists are accurate, then beginning in 1983, doctors should expect to see more patients with skin cancer.

This biometeorologic discovery could have immediate application. It would be easy for doctors and weathermen to inform the public of those years when sunspots are at a raging high. We could either spend less time sunning ourselves during these critical summers, or wear more protective clothes. To help sunbathers get the darkest, safest tan, manufacturers could promote their creams, lotions, and oils containing the least amount of paba (the best sun shield) during the years of minimum sunspots, and their strongest paba preparations (the most expensive) during the dangerous years. And aside from reducing skin damage due to ultraviolet sunlight, the discovery could offer advertisers a new gimmick: eleven-year-cycle ad campaigns.

Under the Weather

Many of the anticipated breakthroughs in biometeorology are going to sound surprisingly like astrological pronouncements. Perhaps we should expect this, since both the science of biometeorology and the art of astrology cover the same terrain — man and the environment. But there the similarities end. Biometeorologic discoveries will be grounded in solid research. One new aspect of that research concerns the role of "weather phases" on daily life.

Your Birth

In a government report entitled "Climate and Health" scientists at the National Oceanic and Atmospheric Administration unhesitatingly state: "The precise date and hour of your birth were determined by the weather." They explain that the end of a normal human pregnancy can fall within about plus or minus ten days of the anticipated birthdate. If your doctor doesn't induce labor, weather conditions will. Statistical studies have confirmed that labor most often starts on days when the temperature rises, barometric pressure stabilizes, and (believe it or not) there is high cloud cover. Birth occurs when "moist air gets into the lower layers, pressure falls, clouds thicken, precipitation [may begin], and winds pick up." NOAA scientists still can't explain how certain weather conditions conspire to induce labor and birth, but they assert that the statistical evidence (from several studies) is so strong that the correlations cannot be ignored.

Your Death

So critical are particular combinations of weather variables on our health that government biometeorologists have divided the complex totality of weather conditions into six phases that seem to account for certain behavioral changes and physical ailments. Women go into labor in phase 3, and birth occurs under phase 4 conditions. Ulcers bleed more and migraines peak in phase 4 weather. Heart attacks reach a high in the transition from 3 to 4 and ebb in phase 1 (cool temperatures, high pressures, few clouds, and moderate winds) and phase 6 (falling temperature and humidity, rising pressure, diminishing cloud cover). Spasmodic diseases of the muscles are aggravated by phase 6 weather. Phase 2 weather (clear, beautiful skies, high pressure, and little wind) "stimulates the body very little," claim NOAA scientists, but turbulent phase 5 weather (precipitation accompanied by cold, gusty winds, rapidly rising pressure, and falling humidity) tends to make us irritable and weaken our resistance to colds and flu. And the life-giving phase 3 to 4 transition apparently follows us to the grave: most deaths occur during this phase change. NOAA scientists suggest that it's erroneous to think of a particular phase as characterizing an entire day's weather; rather, any day can contain several different phases.

Your Behavior

Biometeorologists are learning that weather affects not only our physical health, birth, and death, but also our moods and behavior. Although this connection is far more difficult to establish, they have compiled convincing statistics. Suicides peak during phase 3 weather; so do learning problems among schoolchildren. In the latter case, discomfort caused by phase 3 weather conditions is believed to be one factor; the others remain unknown. The behavioral effects of storms are also being studied by NOAA scientists. In many storm fronts, low frequency magnetic waves are present in large numbers, and human reaction times are slowed if a storm's magnetic frequencies lie between one to six cycles per second — the brain's own sleepy rhythms. Can a storm's magnetism combine with the brain's electromagnetic fields to affect our state of consciousness? Ongoing research should soon answer that question. (See *Ions for Your Health*, p. 161; and *Fields to Modify Your Behavior*, p. 165.)

In 1978 Dr. E. Fuller Torrey published a study on "seasonal schizophrenia" in the *Archives of Psychiatry*. He documented the fact that people born in March and April are more likely to become schizophrenic than those born at any other time of year. Split personality, hallucinations, delusions, and withdrawal from reality are all symptoms that fall under the schizophrenia rubric. Translated into astrological terms, Torrey found that an astonishing number of people diagnosed or hospitalized as schizophrenics are born under the zodiac signs of Pisces, Aries, and Taurus. Torrey is not sure why, but scientists at the National Institute of Mental Health have discovered that the brain's production of two major chemicals implicated in depression and mania — norepinephrine and serotonin — vary with the seasons: norekinephrine peaks in January and July and bottoms out in May and October; serotonin runs through the reverse cycle. May and October happen to be the months in which the greatest number of suicides occur.

According to a recent study, fraternal twins (twins that develop from two separately fertilized eggs instead of one) are born more frequently in spring and autumn than in summer or winter. Does that mean seasonal conditions affect ovulation, sperm production, and fertilization? Biometeorologists are presently at a loss for biological explanations to support their statistical evidence. In fact, at this early stage biometeorology is basically a statistical science.

Expect halting progress in biometeorology, because it's difficult to establish causative links between a set of weather conditions and a human ailment or behavior pattern. But biometeorology is clearly a medical wave of the future. Our ancestors blamed plagues, poor health, and irritable moods on the weather. What we are going to learn in the next two decades may prove them right on several counts. To feel "under the weather" is more than a figurative expression.

Ions for Your Health

There are health standards for indoor temperature and humidity levels and an index for the quality of air outside. By 1990 we may have recommended standards on the ratio of negative-to-positive ions in the atmosphere of office buildings, hospitals, and homes. Pleasanter dispositions, fewer colds, increased vigor, and accelerated rates of healing represent a few of the possible advantages.

The benefits of small air ions were so exaggerated in the

1950s — and totally unfounded, considering the research at that time — that the government put an end to the sale of so-called ion generators, which were supposed to cure every ill from corns to cancer. Due to this adamant stand, serious scientific work on ions was abandoned. It has taken more than twenty years for ion research to recover. Today, it is gaining acceptance and respect because of tightly controlled experiments and because scientists have discovered one important mechanism that explains how air ions may work their miracles.

Air ions are molecules of ordinary air that have taken on a negative or positive charge. They are naturally produced by cosmic-ray showers, by frictional forces in strong winds, and by the shearing of water molecules in waterfalls and in pounding ocean waves. In the laboratory, ions are most commonly produced by an abrupt discharge of electric current into a chamber of air.

But what do ions do?

Anecdotal evidence suggests that an abundance of positive ions causes irritability and nervousness, and more negative ions have a tranquilizing effect. Hippocrates observed that "northern winds occasion disorder and sickness." Winds like the foehn of Germany, the mistral of France, the sirocco of Italy, the *zonda* of Argentina, and the Santa Ana of California carry an abundance of positive ions. Weather-sensitive people assert they can sense the wind hours before it hits, when they experience labored breathing, nervousness, and headaches. In the early 1960s scientists at the Israel Institute of Technology studied the ill winds of Israel, known as the *sharav*. They found that twelve hours before meteorological equipment detected the rise in temperature and drop in humidity that herald the approach of the *sharav*, the ratio of positive-to-negative ions in the air rose.

Most of the evidence we have about ions comes from plant and animal research. The results show that ions produce many different effects:

• Dr. Albert Krueger, a bacteriologist at the University of California at Berkeley and a pioneer in ion research, learned that barley, oat, lettuce, and pea plants grow faster in air enriched with either positive *or* negative ions. These plants are larger and heavier than plants nurtured in ordinary air. Krueger's theory is that air ions speed up biochemical reactions in plants that depend on iron; this helps the plant breathe better and thus grow faster.

• Silkworms thrive on both positive and negative ions. Krueger learned that in ion-fortified air silkworm eggs hatch sooner and larvae grow faster and begin spinning cocoons at an earlier age. When completed, the cocoons are heavier than normal.

• Higher up the evolutionary scale, however, positive and negative ions begin to assume Jekyll and Hyde roles. In rabbits, Krueger discovered that negative ions increase the amount of oxygen absorbed into the lungs and protect tissues in the respiratory tract from infection. Positive ions produce opposite effects.

• Mice infected with flue virus have a better chance to survive respiratory complications if they are allowed to recuperate in chambers containing high concentrations of negative ions.

• Emotions and learning are also affected by ions. Scientists at Pennsylvania State University have documented that the anxiety of rats frequently shocked with electric current is dramatically reduced when the animals breathe air enriched with negative ions. The ions act like a tranquilizer. Other researchers have discovered that, given a choice between negatively charged or positively charged environments, animals prefer to set up house in the negative-ion atmosphere. Scientists at the Battelle Memorial Institute in Columbus, Ohio, showed that rats make fewer errors in learning to run through a maze when the air contains more negative than positive ions.

• One of the few tightly controlled human studies with ions has been done at the University of Pennsylvania. Over 200 burn patients were placed in rooms rich in negative ions. In most cases their wounds dried and healed faster, with less scarring. Even the most severely burned patients felt better, and in 85 percent of these cases negative-ion therapy obviated the need for painkilling drugs.

A Hormone Link

Negative ions do produce beneficial effects, but how? A decade or two may pass before all the intricate links are discovered, but one major breakthrough has already occurred. Scientists have established that positive ions cause the release of serotonin into the blood; negative ions decrease the amount of serotonin in the blood. Serotonin, as we know, is a neurotransmitter, a chemical that relays messages from one brain neuron to another, and plays a role in metabolism, in the relief of pain and anxiety, and in triggering sleep. Krueger has discovered that the adverse effects of positive ions on animals — diarrhea, muscle spasms, and labored breathing — can be duplicated perfectly by an intravenous injection of serotonin. On the other hand, an injection of the drug reserpine, which reduces the amount of serotonin in the body, duplicates the beneficial effects of negative ions. This discovery appears to offer the first biochemical explanation of how negative ions decrease anxiety in electrically shocked rats, and permit burn patients to abandon painkilling drugs. Although negative-ion therapy has yet to be tried on cancer patients, it may offer considerable relief from the disease's excruciating pain.

What can a negative-ion generator in your office or bedroom do for you?

Judging by the anecdotal evidence, such devices are particularly alluring. People in government and business offices who have installed negative-ion generators to remedy stale air, claim they feel invigorated, spirited, suffer fewer colds, and work more efficiently. But the effects of ions on people are just beginning to be investigated under rigorous conditions. Experiments in progress at three universities are examining the potential advantages of negative-ion exposure, and measuring subjects' blood-serotonin levels. Sheelah Sigel, a psychologist who works with Krueger, has been conducting tests with male patients and reports preliminary results that are consistent with animal studies on relief of anxiety and pain. "We are being very cautious about findings," she admits. "We don't want to start another ion craze."

Sigel offers an explanation as to why animals and people should be sensitive to ions. During early evolution, single-celled animals were in direct contact with their environment. As bodies developed, internal cells lost contact with the outside environment, and consequently the nervous system developed to convey external stimuli to these isolated cells. Hormones like serotonin are a major part of this relay system and inform the body of what's happening in the outside world. Ions, Sigel believes, may be one of many environmental factors that affect hormone levels.

We should start to learn the results of ion experiments with people some time in the mid 1980s. If they indicate, as clearly as the animal research does, that negative ions provide definite benefits, ion generators could become as standard a home and office feature as air conditioners. There are, of course, generators on the market now. Their quality, according to researchers, varies widely. Government standards have not been set for ionizers, because not even the most qualified researchers know exactly how ions affect people or what ion concentrations may be required for desirable effects.

Fields to Modify Your Behavior

Breakthroughs to aid you in sharp thinking, fast reactions, and restful sleep should be coming within the next twenty years — not as a result of drugs, but from exposure to small doses of very weak electric fields.

The earth is sheathed in an electromagnetic field, and additional electromagnetic bombardment emanates from radio, television, and electric machinery. We, too, are clothed in a tightly woven cocoon of pulsating biofields. In the past there has been much speculation — and too little solid research — as to how our natural body fields interact with those fields in our environment. Many scientists are now investigating the question.

At the Brain Research Institute in Los Angeles, Dr. W. Ross Adey has demonstrated that ambient electric fields with one-twentieth the voltage of a transmitter battery can affect the behavior of animals. Monkeys and cats were taught to perform a certain task in a given period of time. Then a low-frequency field was introduced into their environment, with the result that the animals performed the learned task more quickly; a slightly different frequency slowed the animals' performance. In other tests, animals — and several people — exposed to field frequencies between seven to ten cycles per second became so relaxed they fell asleep. (The U.S. research with ambient fields is different from the Russian technique of Electrosleep, in which three electrodes are connected to the head — two near the eyes and one behind the skull — and a small current is passed through the brain. It induces sleep that appears to be identical with natural sleep. But there is no evidence that it helps migraine and asthma sufferers, schizophrenics, or palliates the palsy of patients with Parkinson's disease — some of the benefits attributed to Electrosleep.)

The Male Factor

Recent evidence that external electric fields may influence body hormones comes from the work of Dr. H. B. Graves at Pennsylvania State University. He determined that newborn chicks exposed to electric fields grew faster and weighed 10 percent more than chicks in a normal environment. What implicates a hormone — Graves believes it is testosterone — in this case is that only male chicks experienced accelerated growth. Research with mice has also shown that only males grow faster in electric fields.

The effect continues for about five weeks, and then, for reasons still unknown, the fields cease to exert an influence.

The idea that external electromagnetic fields may affect us harks back to the 1950s with the work of Yale University's Dr. Harold Burr. Burr conducted a year-long test with women college students in which he measured their electromagnetic fields daily, using electrodes placed near, but not on, their bodies. Each woman registered small daily fluctuations, and once a month produced a huge jump in voltage that correlated directly with her ovulation. Encouraged by this discovery, Burr studied the fields of 1000 women at New York's Bellevue Hospital. In 102 cases he charted abnormal voltage gradients when he made measurements between the abdomen and the cervix. Medical examinations of these women showed that ninety-five of them had cancer of either the cervix or the uterus.

The discovery that our biofields extend beyond our skin is contributing to a whole new branch of diagnostic medicine. (See *Diagnosing with Magnetic Fields*, p. 227.) It also suggests that our fields may couple with fields in the environment. The combination could have enormous ramifications for our health and well-being. Very weak electric fields, similar to those utilized by Adey, are generated by many kinds of industrial machinery. Power lines also generate these fields out to distances of several hundred yards. Even such weak fields could seriously endanger the safety of industrial workers by slowing down their reaction time.

It is likely that electrical fields affect the brain through entrainment; that is, a field is either synchronized with a brainwave frequency and links up with it, or it is some multiple of the brain's frequencies and couples with them to increase or decrease the brain's energy. Adey believes that eventually certain external electric fields may be used in operating rooms, on board planes and spacecraft, and in factories to sharpen our attentiveness and reaction time. This could have a direct bearing on our learning ability and memory. One of the earliest applications, Adey asserts, could be electric blankets that not only keep us warm, but lull us to sleep.

Light on Your Health

How should you light your home to promote better health and a sense of well-being? What kinds of lights should be installed in windowless offices to provide all the benefits of natural sunlight? By 1985 we may have the answers to these questions from the International Committee on Illumination. Their guidelines may include types of indoor illumination that could influence our body's metabolism, and affect our behavior. The long-awaited recommendations could be of particular importance to schoolchildren, office workers, and the sick and the elderly who spend a good portion of their day in artificial light.

Photobiologists constitute a relatively new breed of scientists; they study the effects of artificial light on animals and people. One of their ultimate goals is to improve the quality of artificial light in which we all spend between a third to a half of our lives. The starting point for their research was the realization that ordinary light bulbs and fluorescent tubes emit what is called a deprived spectrum — these lights lack certain vital ultraviolet rays that exist in ordinary sunlight.

Dr. Richard Wurtman of the Massachusetts Institute of Technology has found that elderly people in nursing homes produce more vitamin D_3, and their bodies use it more efficiently, when ordinary light bulbs are replaced with bulbs that closely simulate the sun's full spectrum. There is evidence, though not yet conclusive, that hyperactivity in children may be aggravated by deprived-spectrum bulbs. Other photobiologists have shown that artificial light can dramatically influence animal behavior. In laboratories, mice and hamsters kept under fluorescent tubes became aggressive; in zoos, birds that refused to mate, snakes and turtles that were starving themselves to death, and fish that were infertile, all adopted normal behavior when ordinary lights were replaced with full-spectrum lights.

The Sex Factor

Scientists are just beginning to understand how light affects animals and people. Dr. Wurtman has found that light striking the photoreceptors in the eye sends a signal to the pineal gland, at the base of the brain. This gland, in turn, secretes the hormone melatonin, which triggers a chain of reactions that play vital roles in health and sexual maturation in animals — and apparently in people, as well. A study of thirty adult women blind since early childhood showed that only two had regular menses. Even women blinded in adult life suddenly shift from regular to erratic menstrual periods. Studies of men blinded before and after puberty also illustrate a direct relationship between the degree of light falling on the retina and the onset of puberty.

Like food, air, and water, sunlight is essential to our survival.

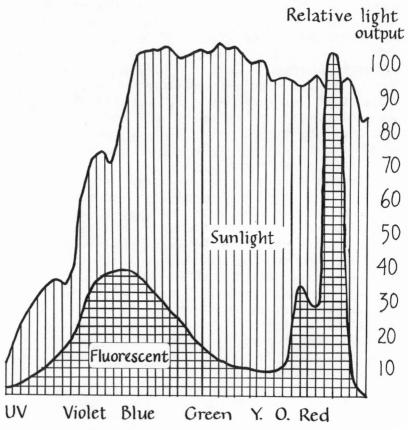

Relative light output

100
90
80
70
60
50
40
30
20
10

Sunlight

Fluorescent

UV Violet Blue Green Y. O. Red

A Deprived Spectrum

These two curves compare the spectrum of natural sunlight with the light emitted from an ordinary fluorescent, or cool white, bulb. Animals reared under such "deprived spectrum" light, in laboratories and zoos, become aggressive, refuse to mate, and have been known to starve themselves to death. People in nursing homes produce more vitamin D3, and their bodies use it more efficiently, when ordinary light bulbs are replaced with bulbs that closely simulate the sun's spectrum. We may soon have federally recommended standards for the kinds of lighting in homes, offices, hospitals, and schools.

Life developed for millions of years under sunlight. It was only ninety years ago that the light bulb was invented and we entered a new era of indoor living. The deleterious effects of this deprived-spectrum living have been widely studied in Russia. Russian law now requires that every coal miner take a daily dose of ultraviolet light; the belief is that this helps prevent black lung disease, caused from inhaling coal dust. Preliminary American experiments with hamsters indicate the treatment works. Russian scientists also report that a little bit of ultraviolet light added to classroom bulbs reduces the incidence of colds in schoolchildren by 30 percent. Exploring that possibility, Cornell University photobiologists are learning that the addition of ultraviolet light also improves visual acuity and evidently reduces fatigue among schoolchildren.

Most of the findings on the effects of light on us are tentative and must be confirmed by additional laboratory research. Yet the evidence amassed from animal studies is so compelling that for the last few years a special committee of the International Commission on Illumination has been collecting and evaluating photobiology research from scientists around the world. One of their recommendations may be the use of full-spectrum bulbs (like Vita-Lite, produced by the Duro-Test Corporation, a New Jersey firm) in hospitals, schools, and nursing homes; for it seems that children, the sick, and the elderly are particularly photosensitive. Relegated to occasional use might be the popular red and pink bulbs. Though they seem to create a sensual, romantic atmosphere, animals exposed to them for prolonged periods of time become restless, irritable, and pugnacious.

16

Earth Breakthroughs:
Predicting Tomorrow's Catastrophes

Forecasting Earthquakes

The promise of forecasting earthquakes has been around for awhile, but at last the ability to predict this most menacing of natural phenomena seems more certain. There are many factors responsible for the change.

We know that the earth's land masses move on about a half-dozen giant plates that often pull apart, scrape against each other, or collide, causing stresses within the rock beneath the earth's surface. When these stresses become too formidable, the rocks slip. If the slippage occurs gradually, the stress is harmlessly vented. If slippage occurs suddenly, however, the earth shudders and a quake results. That, according to geologists, is the basic "why" and "how" of quakes.

The "when" is a harder question to answer. Nonetheless, scientists are uncovering many new clues. The electrical resistance of rocks under pressure varies with stress, and the variation can now be accurately measured and read as a warning signal. Another precursor is the release of gas trapped in the crystal lattice of a rock. The more the cracking increases, the faster the rate of gas diffusion from the rock. Japanese seismologists have charted a high correlation between major tremors and the premonitory presence of helium, nitrogen, and argon gases. A third promising early-warning sign may turn out to be the eerie "earthquake lights," the luminous flares that light the sky hours or days before a quake occurs. Dr. John Derr, a geologist, discovered that earthquake lights have been observed for years by the Chinese and Japanese, that mention of them is even included in an ancient Japanese haiku: "The earth speaks softly to the mountain / Which trembles / And lights the sky."

In earthquake-prone Japan, observers have noted that during several quakes in this century, the sky lit up as if by sheets of lightning, and at times auroral streamers, beams, and fireballs could be seen as far as seventy miles away. More recently, American scientists have reported lights in the sky before and during the 1969 quake at Santa Rosa, California. And the tragic July 1976 China quake generated such intense light that people actually awakened, thinking their lights had been turned on. Physicist David Finkelstein of New York's Yeshiva University has offered one theory for the light phenomenon. He believes that years of stress build up high electrical potential in quartz rocks and that before a quake the current is discharged in the form of lightning. To measure effectively any of these precursory phenomena of course requires massive deployment of measuring devices, and that is precisely the strategy scientists are planning to use in the 1980s and 1990s.

Animal Forecasters

Strangely enough, animals may prove to be the most reliable forecasters of impending quakes.

At the Stanford Outdoor Primate Facility — adjacent, coincidentally, to the San Andreas fault — Dr. Helena Kraemer has observed chimpanzees before earth tremors and thinks she has amassed "the first scientific evidence there are behavior changes that precede earthquakes." Prior to a swarm of minor quakes in June 1976, scientists at the facility noticed that "the animals were more restless and spent more time on the ground than high on their climbing structures and in their nesting areas. Their behavior change was so significant it seems unlikely it was due to chance."

At that time the animals' behavior was recorded, however, the scientists were involved in work unrelated to earthquake prediction and were unaware that any tremors had occurred. It was only in going back over their records to find some cause for the abnormal behavior that Dr. Kraemer realized the chimpanzees' behavior changed markedly on the day before two of the largest tremors that month. A year later a quake rumbled through the

Little Lake Valley area, northwest of San Francisco. A team of animal behaviorists headed by University of California's Dale Lott later interviewed the area's 3000 residents about any unusual behavior in their pets or farm animals. Many animals had remained calm in the twenty-four hours prior to the quake, but others seemed to sense impending danger. Horses kicked their stalls, dogs and cats howled and meowed almost continually and sought the company of their owners, and some animals refused to wander outside their shelters.

What is it animals may sense that warns them of impending quakes?

German biochemist Dr. Helmut Tributsch of the Max Planck Institute in Munich has proposed what many scientists consider the most plausible explanation as to how animals may augur quakes: they sense electrically charged particles in the air that are produced by currents in the earth preceding quakes. These may be the same particles — positive air ions — that precede electrical storms, causing sensitized people to develop headaches, nausea, and irritability. (See *Ions for Your Health*, p. 161.) Studying reports by villagers who survived the Friuli quake in Italy in May 1976, Dr. Tributsch compiled these observations:

Deer formed flocks . . . cats left the houses and the village; at the time of the quake no cat was apparently left in the village. In three cases, cats dragged kittens outdoors and bedded them in green vegetation . . . mice and rats left their hiding places; on one farm mice and rats were observed running around before the quake . . . Fowl refused to roost a few hours before the quake . . . Cattle panicked in their barns; cattle showed clear signs of fear 15–20 minutes before the quake. The animals started to bellow, tear at their chains and paw their boxes . . . Dogs barked without apparent reason 20 minutes before the quake. Some people were guarding their property — suspecting intruders — just before the quake hit.

The Chinese are already depending on animals as an aid to prediction. "Documentation in China is very good," says Dr. John Logan of the Center for Tectonophysics at Texas A & M University. "So is the work done with animals in Japan, Italy and Guatemala." "It is easy and simple to use animals to predict earthquakes," states an overly optimistic report from the seismological station in Tientsin. The report then goes on to supply these clues: cattle, sheep, mules, and horses do not enter corrals; rats flee their homes; hibernating snakes abandon burrows; pigeons take to the air and do not return to their nests; fish leap above the

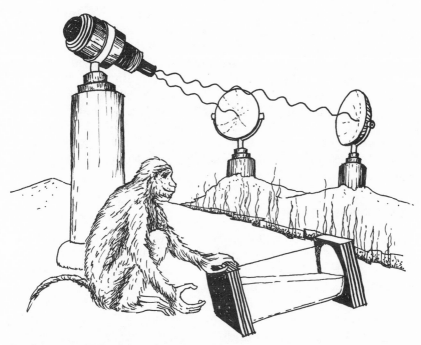

Deploying a Multitude of Detectors

To forecast earthquakes, scientists will rely on new devices — and on animals — to detect many of the precursory phenomena of quakes. Laser beams are bounced off reflectors to record slight elevations in the level of the ground; tiltmeters act like giant carpenters' levels to detect minute tilts in the land; electrically charged particles (air ions), and gases released from fissures deep within the earth, seem to alert animals of impending quakes. Hidden television cameras may soon be used to monitor the behavior of chimpanzees, hamsters, and rats for telltale signs that augur a quake. The new practice in earthquake prediction is to deploy many detectors in the hope that one or more of them will prove sensitive enough to act as an early-warning system.

water surface; and rabbits raise their ears and jump aimlessly up and down.

U.S. scientists suspect that much of the Chinese advice is based on folklore, but Logan and many others predict that some animals more than others instinctively detect the atmospheric changes that herald a quake. The ability of birds to detect magnetic variations, polarized light, and slight changes in atmospheric pressure may make them particularly sensitive to impending quakes — and the best equipped to flee them. "We would be remiss if we did not make some effort to build up scientific evidence to confirm or reject theories about animal behavior and quake prediction," advises one geophysicist.

Several U.S. laboratories are now working with various animals, videotaping their behavior and attempting to correlate it with seismographic readings. In addition to chimpanzees, hamsters and rats have also given accurate warning of quake tremors. Scientists foresee the day when animals will be kept in cages in quake-prone areas. Their actions will be continuously monitored by TV cameras and the tapes scanned by computers for telltale behavioral quirks.

Tidal-Wave Prediction

Tidal-wave, or tsunami (tsoo nah'me), prediction is not as glamorous a field of research as earthquake prediction, but the stakes are still high. A large earthquake, the most common cause of tsunamis, in one part of the Pacific can create waves capable of inundating coastal villages and cities as far away as North and South America, Asia, and the islands in between.

A tsunami — the Japanese word for tidal wave, which has come into international use — moves quite predictably across the open ocean at speeds up to 500 miles an hour. Less predictable, however, is the height the wave may reach before it breaks over a beach or an island, wreaking havoc and death. In 1887 a tidal wave killed more than 900,000 people in China. In 1960 one destroyed or severely damaged nearly every town along 500 miles of the Chilean coast. And as recently as 1974, more than 2500 people were killed by a tidal wave in Bangladesh.

In order to minimize the impact of these killer waves, the thirty-year-old Tsunami Warning System, a cooperative international organization operated by the U.S. Weather Service, is about to be armed with improvements that could save hundreds of thousands of lives. The present system, a network of stations established in 1948, is designed to locate and measure large earthquakes that may create tidal waves, as well as to detect the wave and follow its building front across miles of ocean. The system consists of seismographs and tide gauges that are installed throughout the Pacific and linked to the warning center in Hawaii.

If an undersea quake appears from seismological data to be large enough to cause a tsunami, a watch is issued, alerting threatened populations to the possibility that a tsunami may be in the making. If a wave is actually detected by the tide gauges in the system, a warning is then issued. But because most watches, and many warnings, are not followed by destructive tsunamis, far too often the present system is considered not much more reliable than the unfortunate boy who cried wolf.

Refinements in theory and equipment are forthcoming, however. James Brune of the University of California at La Jolla and Hiroo Kanamori of the California Institute of Technology assert that only very long seismographic waves called 100-second waves are likely to trigger dangerous tsunamis. To test their theory, three very-long-wavelength seismographs were set up in 1978 under a joint Soviet-American program; one in Hawaii, one in Alaska, and the third on the Soviet island of Yuzhno-Sakhalinsk. And others are planned throughout the Pacific. An alarm reading on one or more of the new devices, scientists feel, will provide a fairly good indication that a village or island should be alerted, if not evacuated, once tide gauges detect a crescendoing wave.

Another problem with the present system is time delays. It usually takes up to two hours to relay information from one remote tidal-wave tracking station to another. This should be remedied, however, in the mid 1980s, when the network of stations will be linked by satellites so that information can be exchanged instantaneously and around the clock.

Earth's Methane Core

There is a growing consensus among geologists that tsunamis may be caused not only by earthquakes, but also by methane gas escaping from deep within the earth. One day helicopters equipped with chemical "sniffers" may try to locate these methane leaks to predict possible earthquakes and tsunamis, and also to tap the leaks for commercial gas exploitation. Cornell University planetologist Dr. Thomas Gold estimates there may be enough methane in the bowels of the earth to satisfy the world's energy needs for several centuries.

This new image of the earth as possessing a center of methane gas is Gold's provocative notion. He contends that the main source of carbon that existed on the earth's surface throughout geologic times was not from the carbon dioxide vented during volcanic eruptions — as current theory has it — but from methane, trapped inside the earth when it formed 4.6 billion years ago and leaking ever since. Ample evidence exists, argues Gold, of the presence of such methane. Methane is the source of the torchlike flares and explosions that accompany many earthquakes; jets of methane shooting out of the ocean floor during a quake bubble to the surface to cause tsunamis; and a great pocket of trapped methane is what's holding up the chunk of California known as the Palmdale Bulge.

Perhaps the most convincing evidence for large methane leaks comes from the mud volcanoes, seething patches of mud found in the Caribbean, South America, and central Australia that emit flares of gas as a volcano spews out lava. One mud volcano that erupted recently near Baku in the Soviet Union produced flames over a mile high and burned steadily for eight hours. Gold suspects that the strange behavior of animals prior to earthquakes may be due, in part, to their smelling methane liberated by shocks deep in the ground. In order to prove his methane theory, Gold has asked NASA to send into orbit a satellite in the early 1980s to attempt to locate those regions where the earth is leaking methane. The existence of huge methane deposits would not only go a long way to further our understanding of quakes and tsunamis; it may help solve our energy needs for the future.

17

Weather Breakthroughs:
Weather for the 1980s, 1990s, and Beyond

More Accurate Forecasts

When a weatherman of the 1990s predicts three days of glorious sunshine you can be certain it won't rain. Even the 1980s' weathermen will be able to give more reliable forecasts. Satellites that provide instant global weather conditions will improve accuracy. Also, a more comprehensive understanding of the dynamics of earth's atmosphere, and several recently identified links between weather on earth and solar activity, will contribute to more precise forecasting.

Although a wealth of folklore and anecdotal evidence pointed to a physical connection between solar cycles and terrestrial weather patterns, meteorologists had always been reluctant to admit it. Their skepticism was based on the fact that the total solar energy received by the earth doesn't vary by more than 1 percent in any given year, so heat from the sun alone couldn't possibly account for such phenomena as thunderstorms, hurricanes, droughts, and monsoons. They were sure a more powerful mechanism had to drive earth's weather. Meteorologists now think they've pinpointed such a mechanism in the sun's magnetic fields. Soaring out of sunspots and solar storms, these fields sweep across the earth in giant waves, increasing the intensity of cosmic-ray showers. The magnetic field of a typical large sunspot is 8000 times stronger than the earth's own magnetic envelope. The varied ways in which solar magnetism affects weather are just beginning to surface. Here are some of the breakthroughs that will eventually aid weathermen in making accurate forecasts.

Dry Skies

The amount of carbon in tree rings varies with sunspot activity. Studying tree ring records dating back almost three centuries, J. Murray Mitchell of the National Oceanic and Atmospheric Administration discovered a link between the eleven-year sunspot cycle and the likelihood of droughts in central and western parts of the United States. Droughts seem to occur in these regions a year or two after every second wave of sunspot activity ends; the 1978 droughts, for example, followed the sunspots that ebbed in 1976. Why does a drought occur only once every two solar cycles? Mitchell believes it's because the sun's magnetic field, which controls sunspots, reverses after each eleven-year cycle. Hence the conditions of the field responsible for a drought appear once every twenty-two years. What are these conditions? Can they be detected? And what exactly do they do to earth's atmosphere to dry up the sky? Once these questions are answered, Mitchell believes it should be possible to know a few years in advance those areas throughout the world where droughts will occur — and perhaps, with weather-modification techniques, prevent them from happening.

Snow Skies

Historical records indicate that in the past sunspots have vanished for periods lasting up to a hundred years. Climatologists once thought that ancient observers had simply been lax during these periods in recording sunspot activity. But astronomer John Eddy of the National Center for Atmospheric Research wasn't convinced that ancient heaven-watchers were that careless, and he turned for clues to the oldest trees on earth. Analyzing the carbon in three rings dating back 8000 years, Eddy discovered that, for reasons still unknown, the sun occasionally loses its spots. On earth, the consequences are chilling. Deep-sea soil deposits that offer a layered record of centuries of atmospheric conditions indicate that such spotless episodes have been accompanied by years of extreme cold weather and heavy snowfall — not mini-ice ages, however; just long, severe winters. Sunspot activity will almost certainly be suspended in the future — perhaps in our lifetime. Scientists hope that before then they'll have developed techniques to alert them to such sunspot silences and enable them to forecast how long a quiescence will last.

Rain Skies

The sun may drive terrestrial rainstorms. John Wilcox of Stanford University is learning that certain solar magnetic fields that sweep the earth every seven days can, if they are strong enough, decrease the rotation of global air masses, or vorticity, in the atmosphere. Meteorologists know that increased vorticity whips up an existing storm and expands its outer edge southward, where it picks up additional moisture that can fall as rain or snow in higher latitudes. Wilcox is constructing models to understand how decreased vorticity, caused by solar magnetism, influences clear skies. Fluctuations in the seven-day fields may turn out to be reliable indicators of a brewing storm.

Windy Skies

Solar flares are the most dramatic events on the sun. Intense bursts of energy, lasting from a few minutes to several hours, they gush across space and disrupt radio communications on earth. (If the energy in a typical flare could be harnessed, it would provide enough electric power for the whole world for the next ten million years.) Climatologist J. W. King of England's Appleton Laboratory has discovered strong evidence that these solar flares stir up earth winds. As the sun makes a full rotation on its axis every 27.5 days, the earth is exposed to solar flares of all sizes and strengths. We're aware of the largest ones because they disrupt radio communications, but King claims that even the smallest flares create disturbances in the earth's ionosphere, which influences barometric pressure and wind patterns. Since the effects of a typical solar flare take about two days to reach the earth's outer atmosphere, monitoring the sun's flares would permit meteorologists to predict sudden changes in barometric pressure and wind patterns a day or two before they occur. This capability could do much to increase the accuracy of weather forecasts.

• • •

There is one recent discovery that television and radio weathermen could rely on in making their daily forecasts, but they don't. Several studies have demonstrated that after a solar field sweeps earth, the accuracy of weather forecasts dramatically plunges for the next few days. Magnetic detectors set up around the world show when these sweeps occur and measure their strength. Thus, for a few nights after a sweep a weatherman could simply preface his forecasts with the warning that for a while he is likely to be more inaccurate than usual.

One-Hundred-Year Forecasts

Every event on the sun has an effect on the earth. Past solar flare-ups influenced the formation of our present atmosphere and the evolution of life. Future solar eruptions will influence tomorrow's weather, the growth of crops, and even our health. To understand fully the subtle ways in which the sun fashioned our past — and will shape our future — scientists require a comprehensive and accurate record of the sun's past behavior. Once considered an impossible historical document to obtain, it appears that in no more than a decade we may have a solar record dating back a million years.

Since the amount of the element carbon 14 produced in the atmosphere increases with sunspot activity and solar eruptions, scientists have been able to trace the sun's behavior back 8000 years by studying the traces of carbon in the rings of ancient trees. But our solar system is 4.6 billion years old, so trees obviously don't contain the sun's whole turbulent story.

A more complete record appears to be logged in the earth's massive ice deposits at the North and South poles. Geophysicist Edward Zeller of the University of Kansas has discovered that ice layers formed by eons of snowfalls contain nitrogen compounds whose concentrations rise and fall with recorded solar activity. Analyzing 300-foot plugs of ice from the South Pole, Zeller and his colleagues have already traced the eleven-year sunspot cycle back to A.D. 1150. Samples from Antarctica and Greenland, where ice is more than two miles deep, store a million-year-old solar record.

Zeller is still uncertain whether cosmic-ray activity, which peaks during solar storms, forms the nitrogen compounds, or if they are made by electrical effects in the earth's atmosphere, such as the auroral displays, which intensify with solar eruptions. If tests scheduled for the early 1980s confirm this new nitrogen-dating technique, scientists will begin to chart sunspots, solar flares, and solar winds back to the early days of human life on earth. We may then learn what kind of weather conditions early man had to battle to survive, and how the earth's climate has changed over the last millennium. But most important, a million-year solar record would enable scientists to determine with a greater degree of confidence and accuracy the major weather patterns for the next century and beyond.

Predicting Climatic Disasters

Is the earth heating up, or are we moving into a "little ice age" of the type that produced exceptionally severe winters over much of Europe and North America between 1550 and 1850? Before the end of this century climatologists expect to uncover the answers. They're just beginning to understand the major climatic cycles that have orchestrated past ice ages and warm eras — cycles that will determine as well the earth's weather in the next century, and hence the agricultural production and economies of the nations of the world. One expected breakthrough is the ability to document how significant a factor man has become in transforming the earth's climate.

Climatologists are divided over whether the earth is heating or cooling; there is evidence to support each argument. If it is warming, as the majority believes, we are to blame. Man is guilty of the rise in the atmosphere's level of carbon dioxide because he burns fossil fuels, like coal and oil. In the atmosphere, carbon dioxide acts like a one-way mirror: it allows sunlight to pass through easily on its way to the earth's surface, but prevents heat emitted by the earth from escaping into space. The resulting "greenhouse effect" is warming the world, according to many meteorologists.

A greenhouse warming would wreak havoc on the polar regions. Dr. Stephen Schneider of the National Center for Atmospheric Research recently examined what would happen if the West Antarctic ice sheet loosened and slipped into the sea: ocean levels would rise fifteen to twenty-five feet; Florida's coastal cities would be submerged, as would New Orleans and large portions of coastal Texas, South Carolina, Delaware, and much of New York City and Washington, D.C. "One could launch boats from the steps of the U.S. Capitol," Schneider predicts. Even if flooding didn't occur, the free-floating ice would surely cool the oceans and air currents to such a degree that the earth's weather patterns would be drastically altered. One current study shows that if we continue to burn fossil fuel at the present rate, the atmosphere will be 3° Celsius (5.4° Fahrenheit) warmer by the year 2050 — enough to make Schneider's scenario a reality. This is how warm the earth was 8000 years ago, when many of today's subtropical deserts were swamps and the present-day corn belt of the United States and Canada was parched, barren prairie.

Such drastic events may lie only seventy years away; our own children may live to witness them. Meteorologists warn that the effects of such a warming trend are already occurring: the temperature around large urban areas is warmer today than it was only a decade ago, and over the same period rainfall in urban areas has steadily increased.

Tomorrow's Model

At the Massachusetts Institute of Technology, Ralph Markson has produced a theoretical model of how the atmsophere works that seems to hold real promise for predicting weather and climate. The earth's surface and the uppermost layer of the ionosphere, according to Markson, act as two plates of a capacitor that store electric current. Sunspots and solar flares generate electric particles that ionize the air between the plates; the greater the ionization, the greater the number and severity of thunderstorms and lightning. Environmental pollutants enter this giant electric circuit and, according to Markson's engineering analogy, change the value of global resistances, impedances, and capacities; a climatic disaster is a sort of short circuit, a blown fuse.

The model is very new, but statistics fed into its elegant system of equations provide results consistent with weather patterns. It beautifully explains one recent discovery: shortly after a solar flare eruption, thunderstorm and lightning activity round the world intensifies. Markson's theory will continue to be tested during the 1980s. Scientists consider it the first model that can actually determine how we, through nuclear explosions and environmental pollutants, are influencing weather for the next century.

Are We Entering an Ice Age?

Events on the sun affect day-to-day and year-to-year weather, but very long-term climatic changes like ice ages and global warmings are influenced more by slight variations in the earth's orbit. This 150-year-old theory, advanced by astronomer John Herschel, may soon answer one of the most vital questions in climatic research: When will the next ice age occur?

In 1830 Herschel hypothesized that changes in the orientation of the earth's axis and the shape of its orbit affect the amount of sunlight cast upon the planet. This variation controls the timing

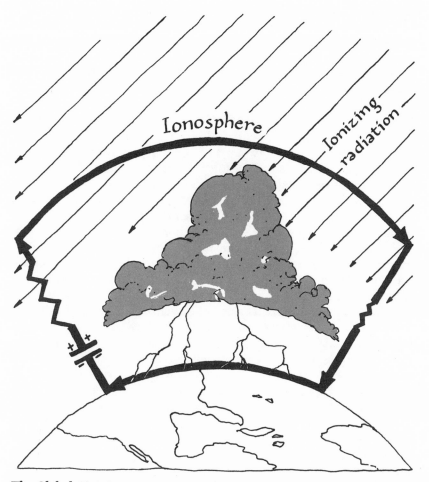

The Global Circuit

The earth and the ionosphere form the inner and outer boundaries of an electrical circuit. Between these two boundaries, the atmosphere acts like a leaky dielectric, a medium that poorly conducts electricity but can sustain electric fields. Ionizing radiation from solar storms influences the circuit — as do environmental pollutants — in ways scientists are just beginning to understand. This global circuit model may allow scientists to predict weather more accurately and to determine how manmade chemicals and radiation from nuclear explosions in the atmosphere affect weather patterns.

of glacial epochs. His theory was long ignored but was revived and augmented in 1941 by Milutin Milankovitch, a Serbian scientist. Today it appears to be the best hope climatologists have for predicting long-range climatic changes. Samples of deep-sea sediment taken from the Atlantic, Pacific, and Indian oceans have confirmed Milankovitch's theory of 23,000-year and 41,000-year climatic cycles for the last 350,000 years. These samples also reveal an unexpected 100,000-year cycle that may be even more important in determining what kind of weather lies ahead.

The earth's axis is currently tilted at an angle of 23.5 degrees. But that angle varies between 22.1 and 24.5 degrees every 41,000 years. The obliquity is known to cause the seasons, and variations in the obliquity strengthen or weaken the contrast between seasons. In addition to its tilt, the axis also precesses, or sweeps out a circle, once every 21,000 years. Precession also affects the contrast between seasons because it determines at what point in the earth's orbit winter and summer occur. Both the 21,000-year cycle and the 41,000-year cycle influence, for example, how much more sunlight Tampa, Florida, receives over Ogunquit, Maine, and what latitudes are best suited for growing rice, corn, or grapes. The recently discovered 100,000-year cycle of extreme cold is still a mystery. The only parameter of earth that changes every 100,000-year cycle of extreme cold is still a mystery. The only parameter of earth that changes every 100,000 years is its eccentricity, or the "ovalness" of earth's orbit. But this eccentricity cycle causes at most a 0.1 percent change in the total sunlight falling on earth — an amount that seems far too small to account for the dramatic 100,000-year cycles of cooling reflected in ocean-sediment records.

James Hays of Columbia University's Lamont-Doherty Geological Observatory is among the many climatologists who are convinced that "changes in the earth's orbital geometry are the fundamental causes of the succession" of ice ages that occurred at intervals ranging from 23,000 to 100,000 years. Small changes in the earth's orbit, says Hays, carry the planet away from the sun, reducing its heat. This chilling is amplified when extra snow and ice, produced by the initial movement, reflect more of the sun's heat away from earth. By this reasoning, Hays predicts that the earth will be moving into a new ice age within 2000 years.

Controlling Weather

In the early 1980s it will be possible to increase accumulations of mountain snow and rain in the High Plains and the Midwest by

10 to 30 percent. By the late 1980s similar accumulations in rainfall will be possible in midwestern farmlands. By the 1990s hurricane winds will be tamed by 10 to 20 percent and crop-damaging hail will be cut by 60 percent.

These predictions were made by the Weather Modification Advisory Board in 1978. They reflect the goals of a major $90 million research effort to control the earth's weather, beginning as early as 1981. After years of promises of weather-modification techniques, it looks as if meteorologists are about ready to deliver. A better understanding of the dynamics of earth's atmosphere, combined with glimpses of how climate is linked to earth's orbital variations and solar activity, has given scientists confidence that their goals can be reached in the near future.

Rain and Snow

Cloud-seeding to enhance rainfall and prevent snowstorms is expected to be the first major breakthrough in weather control. Experiments conducted over the Rocky Mountains have already demonstrated that snow coming from very cold, unstable clouds can be decreased by 54 percent through seeding. So successful were stop-the-snow tests in Colorado that spring flooding from mountain run-off was averted. Tests on lower, more stable clouds are now underway.

It's apparently trickier to make rain than to stop snow. Particles sprinkled into clouds cause condensation of water vapor and hence rain. But scientists are learning that too much seeding is as ineffectual as too little, a fact that has forced them to abandon the "more is better" seeding practice. They're also discovering that rain may fall far beyond the areas seeded. To date, seventy-four countries have undertaken cloud-seeding projects with varying degrees of success. Israeli scientists have achieved the best results, increasing rainfall by 15 percent. American scientists on the WMAB think they can double that amount in parched midwestern farmlands by 1986.

Hurricanes

Trickier still is taming hurricanes by cloud-seeding, which theoretically increases rainfall, thereby robbing a storm of its punch. It's been done but only on a small, play-it-safe scale. So far, tests have been largely conducted in the North Atlantic, where storms normally turn away from land — a necessary precaution in case seeding should intensify a storm. By 1982 scientists hope to have seeded storms in the eastern Pacific, which travel westward away from land. They don't expect to be able to destroy a raging hurricane, but rather hope to subdue its winds by up to 20 percent.

Winter Frosts

Far more ambitious is a plan to prevent winter storms completely. Dr. Krafft Ehricke of Rockwell International has suggested that NASA use space shuttles like the *Enterprise* to lift giant mirrors into orbit around the earth. Ground computers would control the mirrors and reflect portions of sunlight to any spot on earth. Ehricke's mirrors — called solettas, or "little suns" — could be employed to put a quick halt to snowstorms and blizzards, warm frost-endangered orchards, or gradually melt snow with round-the-clock sunlight.

• • •

All these anticipated breakthroughs pose potential hazards, so scientists are, understandably, proceeding cautiously. Recently a plan to seed typhoons in the western Pacific was shelved when nations in the area objected. And the weather-modification report sent to the U.S. Secretary of Commerce in 1978 emphasized the need for international cooperation to avoid actions by one country that would produce adverse weather effects for another. Some scientists believe substantial weather modification is so close to becoming a reality that the nations of the world should begin hammering out an international agreement on the do's and don't's of climate control.

18

Mind-Boggling Breakthroughs:
Strange New Views of Our Physical World

The anticipated breakthroughs discussed in this section — as well as their benefits — are largely intellectual. They stretch our imagination, providing a keener appreciation of our place in creation. These breakthroughs concern the fundamental nature of matter, the forces of nature, and the birth and death of the universe — grand topics that span almost incomprehensible leaps of space and time and imagination. It may be centuries before humankind can benefit from captured quarks or caged antimatter, or engage black holes as sources of limitless power. Several of these topics concern the most profound and universal questions man has dared to ask. The fact that the dilemmas may be finally, and definitively, solved in our lifetime is an awesome and exhilarating prospect.

Black Hole Fever

Efforts to prove conclusively the existence of black holes will reach a frenzied pitch in the 1980s. New equipment is being designed to measure the dribble of energy that spills out of a black hole in the process of digesting a star. Although some scientists feel there won't be conclusive proof of black holes for several decades, their most optimistic colleagues set that date some time before 1990.

Black holes are those mind-boggling gravitational gashes in space where matter has become so dense that light and giant stars are easily sucked in. In a black hole, gravity is so strong that single atoms are mutilated, the laws of physics crumble, and time stops. Little wonder that black holes have captured the imagination of scientists and laymen.

The concept of black holes was advanced in the 1930s but lay dormant until theorists in the 1960s proved that Einstein's equations of general relativity allowed black holes to form from the sudden collapse of very large stars. Since then the search for black holes has been characterized by excitement and controversy. Some physicists think they've already found evidence aplenty of black holes: in the center of developing young galaxies; in the core of quasars; in the constellations Cygnus and Scorpius. And in the galaxy designated M87, which lies sixty-five million light-years away in the constellation Virgo, astronomers are "90 percent certain" they've detected a black hole eating there.

Confusion over conclusive proof is understandable. Matter doesn't fall directly into a black hole but forms a ring, or "accretion disk," around the hole, which steadily feeds it, all the while emitting radiation. It's this dribbling stream of X rays and gamma rays that permits scientists to speculate on the presence of a black hole; indirect evidence at best.

Mini–Black Holes

The image of these holes as entirely black (since not even light could escape) was revised in 1974 by a brilliant British physicist, Stephen Hawking, who illustrated mathematically that atomic particles inside a black hole "tunnel out" until the hole eventually "evaporates." The rate of evaporation accelerates as the hole gets smaller, until the leak is so big and fast-flowing that the black hole, now "glowing," explodes in a flash of energy. This is the most likely fate, asserts Hawking, for a mini–black hole — a mass the size of a mountain compressed into a molehill. Such mini–black holes formed by the billions during the "big bang" creation and are still exploding today with the force of super–atom bombs.

Hawking's theory that black holes radiate is leading to intensified efforts to find them. The space telescope, a ninety-four-inch instrument to be launched in 1982, will be unencumbered by earth's atmosphere as it searches for black holes. Two new X-ray and gamma-ray telescopes will be launched before 1985 to attempt to detect the energy dribbling from mini–black holes. An infrared telescope has been proposed to try to perform the truly spectacular feat of photographing the accretion disk around a black hole, providing positive proof of a black hole's existence. And in New Mexico, the monstrous thirty-by-twenty-mile Very Large Array telescope, consisting of twenty-seven separate dish-shaped antennas, is half-finished and will search for black holes during the late 1980s.

Will the energy of black holes ever be harnessed?

Some physicists have seriously suggested tapping the energy of a mini–black hole in orbit around the earth. A spacecraft would orbit the hole at a safe distance and shoot in chunks of dense matter. As the matter was shredded, it would create radiation that could be converted into microwaves and beamed to earth to serve as raw power for any number of applications. Physicist John Wheeler envisions a space colony just outside the "event horizon," or the rim-of-no-return, of a black hole. The inhabitants would dump their garbage into the hole and collect the radiated energy to power their civilization. Of course, they would have to be careful not to feed the hole too much garbage at one time, or its rim would expand and suck in their colony.

No one can be positive that such grandiose plans will ever materialize, but it may be only a matter of years before black holes have been located to the satisfaction of the scientific community. Theorists are already trying to devise ways to test the first black hole discovered so that they can determine if, as has been suggested, this gravatitional rip in space-time is really a route out of our universe, a dangerous doorway into other worlds whose existence has been depicted only in science fiction.

Gravity Waves

A new generation of observatories will spring up during the 1980s, and though they'll be searching the sky, they won't house telescopes. The new observatories will be designed to detect elusive, ever so subtle, gravity waves. These waves are believed to emanate from cosmic explosions and black holes, and proving their existence is the most difficult challenge facing experimental physicists. The detection of gravity waves would constitute one of the biggest breakthroughs in physics in this half century. Such a triumph would open a new window on the universe — the most exquisitely transparent ever peered through by man or machine.

Gravity waves are one of the more exotic predictions of Einstein's general theory of relativity. They should be produced by an accelerating object, travel at the speed of light, and cause ripples in the very fabric of space-time. Unlike sound, water, or electromagnetic waves, nothing in the universe is immune to the shuddering distortions of gravity waves. Though any accelerating mass (a car, for instance) generates them (and warps the countryside through which it travels), they are so weak that only those produced by the collapse or explosion of a huge star have a chance of being detected.

The first serious attempt to detect gravity waves was begun by Joseph Weber at the University of Maryland in the 1950s. Since vibrations from a passing truck, earth tremors, or a thunderstorm can mask their effect, Weber took extreme precautions. He suspended a large aluminum drum in a vacuum chamber and chilled it to near absolute zero (about −270° centigrade), then attempted to detect minute expansions and contractions as gravity waves from space passed through the drum. Dozens of researchers around the world have followed Weber's example. In 1978 scientists using the world's largest radio telescope, in Arecibo, Puerto Rico, found that two massive objects circling each other 1500 light-years from earth behaved as though they were emitting gravity waves — the strongest evidence yet of the proof of their existence — but the fact remains that after twenty years of excruciatingly tedious investigation, no one is absolutely certain that gravity waves have been detected. Physicists hope soon to rid themselves of that equivocation. During the next decade ingenious new schemes are planned to measure the shudder from gravity waves. This is what we can expect:

• Physicists at the University of Rochester and the University of Moscow intend to use cylinders of niobium (which would be 100 times more sensitive than aluminum), or sapphire and silicon cylinders (which would surpass aluminum by a factor of 1000). Another Soviet team, and scientists at Louisiana State University, hope to use a metal rod with a notch in the center. As gravity waves pass earth, sensitive detectors would measure the fluctuations in the length of the notch. To shield out environmental disturbances, the scientists at Louisiana State University plan to free float their cylinder in a magnetic field.

• Scientists at the California Institute of Technology have proposed a laser "antenna" to detect gravity waves. A beam of laser light would bounce back and forth between the earth and the moon, and measure the slight change in distance between the two bodies as gravity waves rippled by.

• While experimental physicists are setting up their equipment, theorists have already begun to figure out what to expect from cosmic catastrophes. The collapse of stars in our galaxy, the Milky Way, should generate at least one gravitational big event every thirty years; the gobbling up of matter by black holes should produce ten to fifty gravitational extravaganzas a year; and the powerful day-to-day motions of pulsars and binary stars should provide a continuous parade of gravity waves. Hence, if gravity waves exist (and most physicists are convinced they do), they are abundant.

As we enter the 1980s the popular sentiment among physicists is that their new equipment will warp and ripple to the tune of gravity and that this time they'll be able to hear the melody. Once detected and routinely measured, gravity waves will offer physicists their first — and very best — chance to study the internal turmoil at the center of stars, developing galaxies, and black holes. They will be the "television" waves of the universe. Every important event in the cosmos would broadcast a program that could be intercepted and played to a computer for analysis. Gravity waves could provide the most revealing pictures any generation will have of the heavens.

Cosmic Catastrophes

Will the universe expand forever? Will it collapse into another fireball? Was there an actual primordial fireball? Or has the universe always existed?

Just when cosmologists thought they had almost answered these questions (yes, no, yes, no), there is a growing uneasiness among them that perhaps the answers are not as complete as they should be. You may hear a popular cosmologist on a television talk show state flatly that the universe started at a definite moment in time with a big bang and that it will go on expanding until we are spread thin over space. But an increasing number of cosmologists are recommending that we make more room for doubt and humility on these and other "modern" conclusions. The universe may be far stranger than we imagine.

Up in a Puff of Smoke

The most popular cosmologic theory has it that the universe began with the explosion of a primordial fireball 14.5 billion years ago (the most current estimate). The universe has been expanding ever since, as matter scatters and cools. Today there is strong evidence to support this big bang theory, but cosmologists are far less confident about describing the behavior and fate of the expanding universe. If (and it's a big "if") there is a certain critical amount of matter in space, its gravitational pull will one day halt and reverse the expansion; the universe will begin to fall in upon itself, time flowing backward until another fireball is formed and creation begins again. This yo-yo scheme of multiple creations is the fate of a "closed" universe. On the other hand, if there is too little matter to reverse the expansion, the universe is "open," and we will continue spreading through space to become . . . what?

The most recent answer comes from scientists at the University of California at Berkeley. After considering all possible fates of an open universe, John Barrow and Frank Tipler agree with the view of nineteenth-century physicists that an open universe would die a "heat death"; that is, it would lose all organization and pattern and drift into total chaos, a state physicists refer to as maximum entropy. The nineteenth-century physicists arrived at that conclusion based on the laws of thermodynamics, but the California scientists rely on the theory of gravity, and in doing so give the universe's demise a very novel twist. As the universe approaches old age, more and more matter is gobbled up by black holes until the gluttonous creatures begin to regurgitate their meal as showers of subatomic particles. These particles eventually cluster together to form mini–black holes that gorge themselves until they evaporate into pure energy, leaving the universe a sea of radiation. Further, the universe will not expire in its present shape of a sphere. The repeated destruction of black holes and mini–black holes will twist the dying universe into the shape of a long, fat cigar. (Of course, all of this occurs in four dimensions.)

Barrow and Tipler have not answered the question of whether the universe is open or closed, but they have painted a fascinating new picture of THE END — one that nineteenth-century physicists could never have imagined. If the universe is going to suffer a heat death, there seems to be a cosmic rightness to the shape of a cigar.

Is Gravity Weakening?

Imagine a universe in which the laws of physics are forever changing, and where objects on earth fall to the ground more slowly than they did a century ago. The great physicist P. A. M. Dirac developed a mathematical model of such a universe in the 1930s, and, though it's heretical in every postulate, certain aspects of Dirac's model are attracting the serious attention of cosmologists.

Physics and cosmology exist as we know them because of the presence of about a dozen constants: the velocity of light, the mass and charge on an electron, the pull of gravity — to name a few. Empirically determined, these constants are the threads that hold together the most profound equations in science. Interestingly, when two or more of these constants are combined to form dimensionless numbers, the result is either very close to the number one or the huge number 10^{39}. Coincidence? Philosophically minded scientists think not. They view the constants as the missing link between the macrocosm and the microcosm, the long-sought bridge connecting gravitation theory with quantum theory. Intrigued by the physical constants, Dirac found that he was able to construct an amazingly workable theory of the universe based solely on the constants if, ironically, he made one shocking assumption: the gravitational constant, G, decreases as the universe ages. This idea was anathema to physicists, who instinctively felt that certain rules in this ever-changing universe must remain fixed; at least the constants. But today there is evidence that G may, in fact, be decreasing. And since gravity determines the rate at which objects fall, the planets orbit the sun, continents drift apart, and the universe expands, and even influences your body weight, the fact that the effect of gravity may be weakening in no small discovery.

Thomas Van Flanders, an astronomer at the U.S. Naval Observatory, first measured a decrease in G in 1974. He learned that each year the moon pulls another two inches away from the earth and that the tidal forces between the two bodies alone cannot account for the recession. Also, ancient measurements of solar eclipses twenty centuries ago are slightly out of sync with the duration of present eclipses, unless one assumes that G decreases. And geophysicists know that the earth has been expanding since it formed, 4.6 billion years ago, which further suggests that gravity was stronger then than it is now. Though weight watchers wouldn't benefit from such a decrease in gravity — a 150-pound person would grow lighter each year by only about a thousandth of the weight of a potato chip — astrophysicists find Van Flanders' infinitesimal decrease in G (about 7.5×10^{-11} parts per year) fits neatly into those cosmological theories which picture the universe expanding forever. One physicist who agrees with Van Flanders is Vittorio Canuto of NASA's Goddard Institute for Space Studies. "The gravitational constant will continue to decrease forever and the physical conditions of the universe will depart more and more from what they were at the moment when everything started," he says. "Dirac's hypothesis clearly contains the most far-reaching and deepest concepts of evolution."

The final word on G is expected during the late 1980s, when scientists expect to be able to measure the distance between the earth and moon twice as accurately as they can today. If the moon is pulling away from earth faster than it should be, it could mean that gravity is weakening and cosmology is in for a major upheaval.

Antigravity

Instead of the universe crawling at a steady pace to its demise, the universe may be hurtling toward its end. That's the conclusion of Donald Lynden-Bell of the University of Cambridge and William Liller of the Harvard College Observatory. They have found that certain objects in the universe emit radiation that seems to be traveling faster than the speed of light. Rather than contradict Einstein's notion that nothing can exceed the velocity of light, the two scientists consider it more plausible to believe that the illusion of so-called superluminal speeds is created by the universe's expanding faster than we think.

For different reasons, that is also the view of James Gunn of the Hale Observatory and Beatrice Tinsley of Yale University. Their observations of distant objects in space indicate that the universe is expanding faster and faster each year. However, Gunn and Tinsley conclude that an ever-weakening force of gravity may not be the explanation for this acceleration. The phenomenon of accelerated expansion has one shocking implication: since gravity is always an attractive force pulling bodies together, acceleration requires a repulsive force to push galaxies apart; namely, antigravity.

Is there such a wonderful "creature" as antigravity? Very possibly, although scientists don't foresee rocks suddenly floating off into space. If antigravity exists, it would have to be a force that acted only over very long distances and was so weak over a short stretch that its magic could not be displayed. If experiments during the next decade indicate that the expansion of the universe is actually accelerating, scientists will be compelled to determine the cause or causes. If antigravity is the answer, there will be a frenetic race to find the fabulous force, cage it, and ultimately put it to a truly limitless number of tasks. The mere existence of antigravity could make our universe all the more wondrous.

New Creations

There is another threat to the status quo. In a Dirac world, matter must be continually created. A new atom can suddenly appear in the center of a rock and crack its crystal structure. The hypothesis of new matter popping up all over space shocks a lot of physicists, but it hasn't prevented them from searching for new atoms. Scientists are now studying rocks, and if they find what they're searching for, we'll be confronted with an entirely new image of our universe. The philosopher who stated that the only constant is change may yet be right.

Missing Mass

Much of our uncertainty concerning the fate of the universe would be resolved if scientists could only locate the "missing mass." Or — and this is also a possibility — definitely prove that no mass is missing. Within a decade this perplexing fifty-year-old riddle may finally be resolved, and the description of the ultimate fate of the universe will enter the next generation of science textbooks as fact, not speculation.

Gravity is the universe's glue. It holds together solar systems and galaxies. Hence, a major dilemma in cosmology arises from the fact that there doesn't appear to be enough matter in the universe to gravitationally hold everything together. At the great velocities with which galaxies rush through space, they should be flying apart. Yet they're not. So astronomers are forced to conclude that there must be tremendous amounts of matter hidden in space. This missing mass is crucial, because in the general theory of relativity the density of matter determines whether the universe is open and will expand forever, or is closed and will eventually collapse.

Many candidates have been proposed as sources of the missing mass, but the most promising possibility of all appears to be simple galactic gas. X-ray photographs of the sky taken by the Uhuru satellite and just recently analyzed by scientists at the Harvard and Smithsonian Center for Astrophysics pinpoint vast amounts of gas clouds far beyond the Milky Way. Astronomers believe such volumes of hot gas may also exist in other parts of space, and there's even the chance, not all that remote, that enough gas may exist to close the universe. Scientists should have more evidence by 1985, when the Harvard and Smithsonian group expects to have made new observations with the High Energy Astronomy Observatory satellite.

Ironically, news of the hot gas comes just when most astronomers had satisfied themselves that the universe would continue expanding forever, and others figured this expansion was accelerating. It would not be the first time (nor certainly the last) that astronomical observations of the sky produced antithetical views, sending astronomers back to their telescopes. The final word on the missing mass, and thus the verdict on the demise of the universe, may be settled in our lifetime.

Where Are the Quasars?

A new astronomical technique may permit scientists to determine by the mid 1980s whether quasars are bright relics at the edge of the universe, or nearby objects whose brilliant glow is governed by an unknown phenomenon — and thus settle one of the most baffling mysteries in all of modern astronomy.

Discovered in 1960 by Allan Sandage, quasars (quasi-stellar radio objects) are objects that shine with a brilliance 1000 times that of our Milky Way but are only the size of a large star. So anomalous is their fierce glow that astronomers have labored to determine how far away they are and what fires them.

Scientists know that light emitted from any object traveling away from a stationary observer drops in frequency (as does the whistle of a passing train) and reddens in color. This "red shift" is a yardstick, and of all the objects in the universe quasars possess the greatest red shifts. It's wonderful news, on the one hand implying that quasars are the most remote, ancient relics of the universe and hold secrets about creation. But their great distance poses a conundrum: How can any object that far away be so bright? It can't, say some astronomers, so quasars must be close by. Then that means their red shifts are misleading. Yet many astronomers are certain the red shifts are accurate measuring guides.

Baffled, and battling among themselves for two decades, astronomers have searched for a way to determine the real facts about quasars. What they need is a "standard candle" — an object whose inherent brightness can be measured against itself as the object is transported away from the observer. They may soon have it. Scientists at the University of California have discovered that a particular line of light in a quasar's spectrum appears to constitute a true, steady measure of a quasar's intrinsic brightness. Relying on this line as a yardstick, astronomers have already begun to recalculate the distance of quasars, and hope in a few years to locate the quasars and to use their motions to determine whether the expansion of the universe is really slowing down or accelerating, thus solving a significant riddle. This fresh research may also answer another important question: Are quasars young galaxies in the early stage of evolution? If so, they afford a glimpse into our turbulent past.

An Abundance of Antimatter

Our Milky Way galaxy may contain scads of antimatter. Luckily for us, it appears to be caged and at a very safe distance. If this recent astronomical observation is right, scientists may be on the road to explaining the apparent and bewildering absence of antimatter in the universe.

It has been assumed for many years that every particle in nature has an exact opposite, and that the amount of matter in the universe equals the amount of antimatter. That we live in a world dominated almost exclusively by matter suggests to physicists that somewhere in space lurks a massive bulk of antimatter, sufficiently distant not to threaten planets, stars, and galaxies with annihilation. But where is it?

Since the first particles of antimatter were detected in laboratory experiments in the 1930s, many searches of space have uncovered only trickles of the dangerous stuff. Using measurements from a new gamma-ray telescope suspended in a balloon over Australia at 130,000 feet, American scientists were recently led to believe they had located vast amounts of antimatter behaving wildly at the center of our own Milky Way. When particles of matter meet antimatter, they engage in a very brief dance (spinning round each other like subatomic dervishes) and in the process annihilate themselves to produce a pair of vigorous gamma rays of 511,000 volts each. Early calculations indicate that the center of our galaxy is teeming with a trillion trillion trillion million matter-antimatter annihilations every second. Enough violence to make some black holes seem tame.

Physicists are excited and puzzled by the discovery. Why, in our galaxy at least, is all the antimatter concentrated at the center? Is there enough of it to balance the amount of matter in the Milky Way? Is this the remains of antimatter created from the big bang? Some scientists assert the antimatter at the galactic center is new, being continually created. Britain's Stephen Hawking has proposed an exotic explanation: the big bang molded many mini–black holes that continue to this day to exhaust themselves and evaporate, emitting streams of particles and antiparticles. This means that the center of our Milky Way (and probably other galaxies) contains not only annihilating antimatter, but hungry black holes as well. Galactic centers have always been pictured as arenas of violent activity, but now it appears that they may be even more formidable than as depicted in science fiction. Scientists are debating whether antimatter is caged at the center of every galaxy, if that's its favorite spot.

Several gamma-ray observations from balloons are planned during the early 1980s, when scientists will attempt to determine whether antimatter is actually being created anew, and to solve the tantalizing puzzle of why all the antimatter is concentrated in the center of our galaxy. Although the physical cause remains a mystery, we can with certainty say that if the antimatter were not concentrated at the center of our galaxy, we most likely would not be here to ponder its location.

How Galaxies Form

It won't be long before computer simulation of the conditions prevailing in the primeval universe will provide the first pictures of the evolution of galaxies. On a computer's television screen scientists will then watch the birth of our own Milky Way galaxy and formulate how our solar system ended up far out in one spiral arm.

Galaxies are among the most dazzling, majestic, and enigmatic wonders in the heavens. Giant clusters of gas, dust, stars, and planets, they shape themselves into two basic forms, spiral (like our Milky Way) and elliptical. But the forces that choreograph these stellar extravaganzas and keep them kicking are still a mystery. Several years ago Alan Toomre at the Massachusetts Institute of Technology advocated that computers have the promise of re-creating creation itself. Many scientists have responded to this challenge and are working with computer simulations to answer one of cosmology's great riddles: How do galaxies form?

Ellipses

At NASA's Ames Research Center, Richard Miller has developed three-dimensional computer pictures of elliptical galaxies that have astronomers worried. Miller is using the world's largest computer, ILLIAC IV, to learn why certain galaxies take elliptical shapes. He has fed the computer sets of spinning clusters of 100,000 stars and watched them collapse under their mutual gravity. They tumbled into shapes resembling long fat cigars. Since optical observations suggest that elliptical galaxies are shaped more like squat spheres, Miller's results have caused astronomers to take another look through their telescopes. His computer simulations are also creating exotic stages in the formation of galaxies that no one ever dreamed possible. His models begin as spinning spheres of stars, collapse into disks, inflate into smaller spheres, then separate into parallel saucer-shaped plates that eventually fall together and pass *through each other* to end up as fat cigars. Does this bizarre dance represent the true course of the evolution of galaxies? Astronomers are already searching for such strange configurations while Miller continues to refine his images. By spinning spheres of stars at different rates, Miller intends to test the modern belief that elliptical galaxies might have been spiral ones if they had had sufficient spin.

Spirals

Scientists have always assumed that gravity constituted the most likely force behind the formation of galaxies. But researchers at IBM's Watson Research Center have tried an unorthodox approach to galactic formation and are producing excellent results. They programed their computer with the violent life and death story of a giant star. Its ferocious burning during its lifetime generates winds of charged particles and radiation that act like a cosmic tornado to round up debris; death occurs in a huge explosion whose shock waves further corral material into a core in which temperatures rise until it fuses into another star. With this chain-reaction scenario of star cloning star, the computer simulated elaborate spiral galaxies that closely coincided with the facts known about them. Where previous researchers have failed, the IBM team's nongravitational model is the first to produce spiral galaxies whose flailing arms last for about ten billion years, the presumed average age of galaxies. Many cosmologists are disturbed by the success of the nongravitational approach, because it suggests there are other vital, still unknown forces necessary for shaping the cosmos. The IBM scientists do not claim that their model reveals cosmic events as they actually are, but their success in arriving at accurate answers opens up a whole new avenue in exploring creation in the coming decades.

Many galactic mysteries remain to be solved before a complete picture of creation emerges. The tremendous combinative powers of computers to assemble stars by the billions and let them play out their fates is just what is needed for a comprehensive understanding of creation.

The Sun and Planets

Space exploration through the 1980s will continue to involve unmanned voyages to the planets and their satellites. Craft will fly by planets or make soft instrument landings. One will catch up with Halley's Comet when it returns in April 1986, attempting to land an instrument package on the comet's icy head. It's impossible to forecast the countless breakthroughs anticipated in planetary science, but two heavenly bodies, Pluto and the sun, which define the boundaries of our solar system, are sure to be at the center of controversy in the decade ahead. So they deserve particular attention.

The Paradox That Never Was?

Two groups of scientists are rushing to solve one of the most perplexing mysteries about the sun: "The Case of the Missing Neutrinos." When the mystery is solved, we shall finally comprehend one of the major secrets of how stars burn, grow old, and die.

The sun shines because it is a hot nuclear furnace, a fusion bomb that continually converts hydrogen into helium. This protean feat is accomplished through the so-called proton-proton cycle — according to modern solar theory. But if the sun actually generates energy by this reaction (and it's the most plausible choice), then weightless, chargeless, wispy particles called neutrinos should shower the earth in a ceaseless, blanketing rain. But they don't. Traps painstakingly set for over a decade have caught only about one quarter of the neutrinos theory predicts should exist. Solar scientists are nonplused. Where are the missing neutrinos? Or is our current understanding of how the sun shines erroneous? If so, then a good deal of our understanding about the evolution of stars rests on shaky ground.

A team of scientists from the Brookhaven National Laboratory has spent much of the last decade nearly a mile below ground, in a gold mine in South Dakota, trapping neutrinos. They use a 100,000-gallon tank of a common dry-cleaning fluid and work deep underground to shield their equipment from cosmic rays. Their failure to date to detect sufficient quantities of neutrinos, they believe, is due merely to the limitation of their equipment. Neutrinos interact with the cleaner fluid to convert chlorine to argon, but it takes strong neutrinos to do this, and most of the solar neutrinos are apparently very feeble by the time they reach earth.

The Brookhaven scientists think they've solved the problem. During the early part of the 1980s they plan to count neutrinos in fifty-ton tanks of the element gallium, a far more effective trap. Neutrinos convert gallium into radioactive germanium, which is relatively easy to detect, and weak neutrinos can do this. Because the sun is a thick plasma, most radiations generated in its interior require millions of years to fight their way to the surface, then eight minutes more to travel to earth. Thus, we receive extremely dated information about the workings of the sun's internal furnace. Wispy neutrinos, on the other hand, escape to the sun's surface in only three seconds, and eight minutes later hit earth. Neutrino-monitoring, then, is one method that could reveal current events in the core of the sun.

The ability to detect solar neutrinos and monitor their flux could yield unexpected boons. For instance, knowing when the solar furnace is turned up or down could be vital to our understanding of weather and climate. Just a 2 percent drop in solar radiation reaching the earth is considered to be detrimental enough to cause a global ice age. Even a fraction of that change in the sun's energy would decimate crops, diminish rainfall, and result in mass starvation. Ironically, now that neutrino-hunters feel confident that they can bag their game, another group of scientists, swayed by a recent discovery by physicist Henry Hill, are debating whether any neutrinos are, or ever were, missing.

Our Rapidly Cooling Sun

In 1978 Henry Hill of the University of Arizona made a discovery that could qualify as the biggest breakthrough in solar physics in several decades. Hill found that the sun shakes like a giant mountain of jelly. In a physicist's language, the sun appears to oscillate, not in one frequency, like most stars, but in a chorus of frequencies. This produces ripples that push the sun's surface out toward the earth, then every hour or two draw it back. These powerful ripples, Hill theorizes, are gravity waves; if he's right, they would provide a means for scientists to observe the turbulent events occurring at the sun's core. As geophysicists use seismic waves to study the earth's interior, astrophysicists would be able to work with the gravity waves to define the internal structure and behavior of the sun.

Gravity waves could also solve the neutrino paradox. If the waves exist, they could be rapidly transporting large amounts of energy from the sun's interior into space and causing the sun to cool more than a million times faster than current theory allows. A cooler sun means fewer neutrinos: the scant number collected by the Brookhaven team may be all there is. It would also force astrophysicists to reconsider seriously their ideas about the activity on stars smaller and larger than the sun. Independent teams of scientists in the United States, England, and Russia expect to test Hill's theory in the early 1980s. Their results are eagerly, and anxiously, awaited.

There May Be a Ninth Planet

Every schoolchild knows there are nine planets in our solar system. By 1985, however, that number may be reduced to eight, then increased to nine. But the second time around, the ninth planet won't be Pluto.

Astronomer James Christy of the U.S. Naval Observatory has discovered a suspicious lump on one side of Pluto. It may prove fatal to Pluto's status as a planet. Pluto itself would have to be at least six times as long as it is wide to produce the bulge — and such a cigar-shaped planet would soon shatter under the stress of rotation. The most likely interpretation of the lump is that it's a close-orbiting moon. A moon for tiny Pluto spells trouble, for it means the planet is even smaller than anyone estimated. Assuming the bulge is a moon, Christy calculated that Pluto is forty times lighter than current estimates and has a density less than that of water; in short, it's nothing more than a snowball of frozen gases. Some astronomers troubled by Pluto's status have already suggested that Pluto be demoted to a "minor" planet. If Christy's observations prove correct, schoolchildren in the 1980s may well be learning about the sun and the eight planets.

Astronomers, however, won't be certain whether Pluto has a moon until new photos, taken over the next few years, show a clear separation between the planet and its satellite. Meanwhile, Christy has named the moon Charon, after the mythological boatman who ferried souls into the God Pluto's underworld. An interesting fact about Charon is that its orbital period of 6.4 days is the length of the Plutonian day. This means that if Charon is actually a moon, it must hang stationary over one point on Pluto's surface.

Planet X

Two other astronomers at the Naval Observatory — Robert Harrington and Thomas Van Flanders — have proposed a tenth-planet theory to explain the formation of Pluto and its moon. They theorize that in the distant past an unknown planet with a mass three or four times that of earth passed near Neptune and gravitational forces ripped off a chunk of matter that became Pluto. During the close encounter, tidal forces also tore out a piece from Pluto that became its moon. Planet X's own motion was violently disturbed by the near collision, and it was hurled into the darkest reaches of the solar system, where, speculates Harrington, it's probably drifting around, too faint to be seen. Interestingly, in 1972 two astronomers showed that the observed motion of Neptune suggested the existence of an object about two to five earth masses lying beyond Pluto.

Many astronomers are highly skeptical of the existence of a tenth planet, but that has not stopped them from beginning a painstaking search of the sky. Pluto next comes closest to the sun (well within the orbit of Neptune) in 1989. But before that time Pluto may no longer be categorized as a planet, the violent intruder may have been located, and the mysterious tenth planet may in fact turn out to be only the ninth planet after all.

Nature's Building Blocks

Is there a fundamental particle in nature out of which all matter is composed? Or is matter an endless series of seeds within seeds within smaller seeds? To physicists, this 2000-year-old question is the most basic to their science. Many times over the centuries they thought they had solved this conundrum, only to discover later that they had complicated the issue. Well, the answer may be forthcoming within the next two decades. Not only would this constitute the century's biggest breakthrough in physics, but it could drastically alter the way in which we regard all matter.

At the beginning of this century, physicists considered atoms the ultimate and indivisible building blocks of nature. Before the middle of the century, they had changed their minds, for they had delineated the basic building blocks of atoms — electrons, protons, and neutrons. When scientists began colliding these new "elementary" particles head on in accelerators, they unwittingly unleashed at least 200 even "more elementary" particles within a few years' time. This was as exciting a discovery as it was frustrating. Nature seemed to delight in being devious, and the very term "elementary matter" appeared to be a joke.

Currently, many physicists believe that the structure of matter can be ultimately explained by the existence of six kinds of building blocks called quarks. Whimsically named for the properties (quantum numbers) of particles they represent, the six quarks are Up, Down, Strange, Charm, Truth, and Beauty. Quarks are colored, figuratively speaking, red, blue, and yellow, so that certain assortments yield tan gossamerlike neutrinos, and other combinations yield neutral-colored stable particles. This is supposed to be fact, not fiction. Two physicists at the University of Chicago have even suggested that certain combinations of quarks could be manipulated to form stable and very strange gases. What they are labeling "Beauty-Up" gas and "Anti-Beauty [Ugly?]-Up" gas could, supposedly, be safely stored in containers, and minuscule quantities could form a veritable power plant, since mixing just two molecules would result in their annihilation into ten billion volts of pure energy. In their technical report the physicists write: "Stable quarks would, therefore, offer the possibility of storing very high useable energies within small volumes. The technological possibilities are self-evident."

The Quest for Beauty

Quarks are so abstruse that physicist Murray Gell-Mann lifted their name from an equally abstruse phrase in James Joyce's *Finnegans Wake:* "Three quarks for Muster Mark." Having recently uncovered convincing, though indirect, evidence for the existence of five quarks, physicists are pushing their accelerators to the limit to find evidence for the still elusive Beauty. California physicists at the two-mile-long Stanford Linear Accelerator are building a sensitive new detector, Mark III, to search for her (the only creature in physics with a sex) in the early 1980s.

Finding Beauty, though, may not end the game. A new generation of more powerful accelerators will begin appearing in the late 1980s; some of them will make it possible for the first time to collide matter with beams of antimatter. The offspring of these strange unions, some physicists contend, may reveal quarks to be merely another intermediate limb of nature's family tree. Will this regression ever end? Physicists are divided over this dilemma. According to Geoffrey Chew of the University of California, matter has no bottom level; the most definite answer physicists can ever hope to possess is the immutable law that governs the behavior of matter. Theoretician T. D. Lee at Columbia University has solved the riddle by changing the rules of the game. He has proposed a mathematical model that expresses matter not as discrete particles, but as continuous waves called solitons, which by their very nature cannot be subdivided. A still more simple hypothesis is the theory of "nuclear democracy," which holds that all particles created are fundamental.

Despite this uncertain state of affairs, most physicists remain optimistic that, one way or another, they will solve the dilemma soon. If matter has a definable essence — and deep in his or her heart every physicist hopes this is true — finding that essence will permit physicists to erect a new theory of matter anchored to sturdy and permanent foundations. At the moment no one is certain quite what form the theory will take, what new facets of nature it will reveal, or what revolutions in physics it may usher in.

On the other hand, if matter turns out to be infinitely reducible; that is, if every mysterious new particle is just a known particle wearing a different disguise selected from an infinitely diverse and fanciful wardrobe, that news will be greeted more warmly by philosophers than by physicists. Two thousand years ago the Greek philosopher Democritus argued that nature was composed of individual particles called atoms; his opponent, Anaxagoras, claimed that matter consisted of seeds nested in seeds, ad infinitum. We will be supremely fortunate if the ancient riddle is solved in our lifetime.

Supergravity

Einstein spent the last twenty-five years of his life trying to develop a theory that could eventually lead to the unification of the four fundamental forces of nature — gravity, electromagnetism, the weak nuclear, and the strong nuclear. Since then, physicists around the world have tackled this seemingly insurmountable task without real success. Recently, though, there has been cause for renewed optimism among physicists, for it had been demonstrated that two of the four forces are one and the same. And a new theory called supergravity is gaining a lot of attention. It may be precisely the tool physicists need to help them unite nature's remaining "three" forces.

What makes the task of developing a unified field theory extraordinarily difficult is the vast diversity of the force. Gravity is weak and omnipresent, and always has an attractive, or pulling, influence. Like gravity, electromagnetism also acts over long distances, but it's almost infinitely stronger than gravity and can be both attractive (pulling particles together) or repulsive (pushing particles apart). The two extremely short-range forces, the weak nuclear and strong nuclear, usually act solely within atomic nuclei and are always repelling influences. Forces, of course, must influence something, and to the consternation of physicists each of nature's four forces acts on different "things." Gravity affects all matter; electromagnetism manipulates only electrically charged particles; the weak nuclear force acts on electrons, ghost-like neutrinos, and the strangely beautiful and truly charming quarks; the strong nuclear force acts only on quarks. As if this were not confusing enough, even greater diversity exists among these forces. According to modern field theory, forces (or, more properly, interactions) exist because of the exchange of particles. And all four forces exchange different particles. Gravity exchanges within its own ranks the as-yet-undetected gravitons; electromagnetism, photons; the weak nuclear force, creatures called intermediate vector bosons; and the strong nuclear force, gluons, whose name almost speaks for itself. How could any sane person hope to unite forces so vastly and fundamentally different? Why would anyone even think such antithetical forces could be united? The answer is symmetry, an underlying harmony in nature. The human instinct tells us that if we probe deeply enough, we shall observe nature's inherent harmony, no matter how contrasting surface appearances may be.

And Then There Were Three

In the 1960s physicists Steven Weinberg of Harvard and Abdus Salam of London's Imperial College accomplished the first major

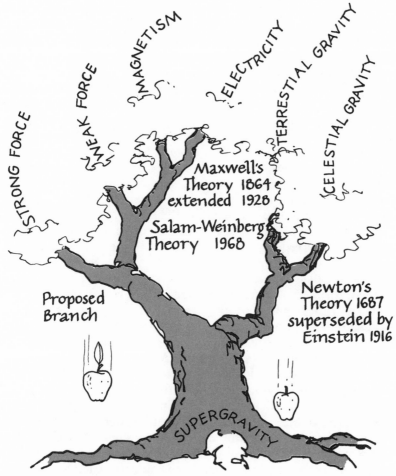

Nature's Family Tree of Forces

Attempts to unite the fundamental forces in nature date back to Newton, who showed that the trajectory of projectiles on earth and the orbits of the planets adhere to the same law. Thus, Newton combined the concepts of celestial and terrestrial gravity. Two centuries later, James Clerk Maxwell proved mathematically that moving electric charges create magnetic fields. He thus established a fundamental relationship between the forces of electricity and magnetism. Einstein's general theory of relativity has superseded Newton's (though not invalidated it), and Maxwell's theory has been extended to form the so-called theory of quantum electrodynamics. In 1968 the weak nuclear force (which operates within nuclei) and electromagnetism were determined to be one and the same. The new theory of supergravity, based on fundamental symmetries in nature between elementary particles, appears to offer the best hope yet of achieving the physicists' dream of a unified field theory.

breakthrough toward unification: they formulated a theory linking the electromagnetic and the weak nuclear forces. In 1978, a crucial experiment at the Stanford Linear Accelerator provided compelling evidence that their theory is accurate. The electromagnetic and weak nuclear forces are fundamentally one and the same — the "electroweak" force, as some physicists have proposed calling the union. If you have trouble comprehending such a dichotomy, imagine how radically different the behavior of a person with a split personality can be. Sybil Dorsett, in the book *Sybil*, is a shy, meek artist with a soft voice and her own preferences in food, clothes, and friends; then suddenly she's Peggy Ann Dorset, a spiteful, violent woman, speaking in a shriller voice, harboring different memories, and displaying her own preferences in food, clothes, and friends. Weinberg and Salam proved, in effect, that Sybil and Peggy Ann share the same brain. Their success has spurred hope that a complete unified field theory is in reach.

Different physicists are taking different approaches. Some experimentalists are searching for gravitons and gluons; experiments with these particles, they think, may suggest the connecting relationships among all particles. Theoreticians, on the other hand, are trying several ingenious mathematical approaches to unite the remaining "three" forces. Supergravity, a mathematically elegant theory and one of the most promising, is based on a newly found "supersymmetry" in nature. This supersymmetry is a complex mathematical property of matter that apparently has always existed but only recently been recognized. It permits physicists for the first time to organize into one family two strangely different classes of particles known as bosoms and ferimons. It's as though some primitive biologist suddenly discovered that, despite their different taste, texture, and appearance, oranges and figs belonged to the same family of foods — fruits — because they contain similar sugars and nutrients. Supergravity has not yet been tested, but in combining several of the most fundamental concepts in modern physics it has already achieved more than any other theory proposed.

The research on supergravity must await the construction of ultra-high-energy accelerators that will begin operation in the early 1990s. Physicists believe that nature's four forces appear to be so different today because the universe is operating at a much lower energy level than at the time of the big bang. As experiments reach higher and higher energies, which, cosmologically speaking, is equivalent to going back in time, the contrasting aspects of these forces should disappear and the harmony that previously existed among them should surface. The 1990s' accelerators could be sufficiently powerful to simulate the conditions of early creation. Strange particles will collide with energies they possessed at the beginning of time. Their behavior will be the most primitive ever observed; their offspring, the Cain and Abel of nature. What we learn from these experiments will have staggering implications not only for physics, but for all of modern cosmology.

Where We Are

Preposterous as it sounds, and despite the statistical evidence against it, the pre-Copernican idea that we are at the center of the universe has regained popularity. Proposed by cosmologist George Ellis of the University of Cape Town, the theory is unacceptably anthropocentric, yet, surprisingly, it does not violate current astronomical observations. Even if it can't be true, we may learn something by imagining ourselves at the center of creation.

Relativity theory permits the possibility of the universe having two "centers" in sort of yin and yang opposition. These eyes in the face of the universe peer unblinkingly, if strangely, from Einstein's equations. In Ellis' model of the universe, we are highly privileged to live in the calm "anticenter"; far across from us at the "center" is a disturbing, unhospitable feature called a naked singularity — a rip in space-time that is continuously pouring new matter into the universe and sucking out old. This hot, dynamic center, says Ellis, is what cosmologists have misinterpreted as the big bang. Creation isn't a one-shot happening; it's a continuing day-to-day occurrence. Ellis has depended on his model to account for various cosmic phenomena, though he never claims his model describes how things are; just how they could be.

Why should we be so lucky as to be at the calm center of the universe? Weren't the odds overwhelmingly against our achieving such a privileged site? Our privileged position is certainly not untenable to those who believe the universe was created for us. Ellis views it the other way round: the conditions most favorable for life are those very near the center, where the universe is cool, calm, and stable. Thus, we are not at the center due to privilege but by accident. And perhaps we constitute the only life in the entire universe.

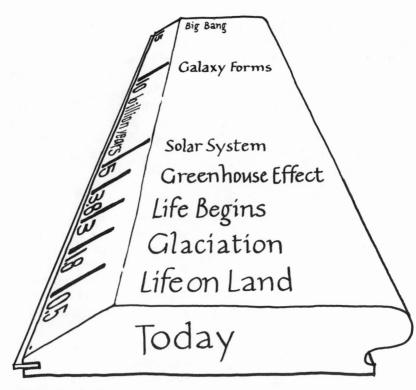

Big Bang

Galaxy Forms

Solar System

Greenhouse Effect

Life Begins

Glaciation

Life on Land

Today

10 billion years 5 3.8 3 1.8 0.5

Life as a Long Shot

Proponents of the "anthropic principle" maintain that the evolution of life is a rare occurrence and that earth may be the only planet in the universe with intelligent beings. Even if earth is not the only outpost of life, new evidence suggests life in the universe may be rarer than scientists expected. It seems that just as life gets started on most planets, it is snuffed out either by the suffocating heat of a greenhouse warming or by rampant glaciation. Life emerged on earth about 3 billion years ago, sandwiched precariously between a greenhouse warming (3.8 billion years ago) and an extensive ice age (1.8 billion years ago).

Are We Alone?

Curiously enough, just when (or because?) so many scientists are searching for evidence of extraterrestrial intelligence (ETI), a number of astronomers and biologists are becoming increasingly vocal about the possibility of the existence of ETI being infinitesimally small. Some have gone so far as to recall the centuries-old notion, now referred to as the "anthropic principle," that we are alone in the universe. "Chances are overwhelming," says physicist John Wheeler, "that the earth is the sole outpost of life in the universe."

The modern-day anthropic principle clearly represents the views of a minority. It's based on recent evidence that the creation of earth's life-giving atmosphere was not one of orderly evolution over 4.6 billion years, but a lucky fluke, an astronomical long shot. The most detailed study undertaken of the evolution of the earth's atmosphere was completed in 1978 by Michael Hart of NASA's Goddard Space Flight Center in Maryland. According to his study, it seems that earth barely escaped two major crises that destroy most life on planets just as it begins. First, the earth almost suffocated 3.8 billion years ago from a runaway greenhouse effect — sunlight trapped in earth's dense atmosphere could not escape. Had the planet been situated five million miles closer to the sun, no oceans would have condensed and a thick hot atmosphere of carbon dioxide, topped with clouds of acid rain, would have formed. This is the current state of the planet Venus.

The second crisis occurred 1.8 billion years ago, when ice spread over more than 10 percent of the earth. The earth came to within only 1° centigrade of pervasive glaciation. Had the planet been 1,240,000 miles farther from the sun, ice would have spread substantially enough to thwart the growth of life. This is similar to the current state of the planet Mars, which may have layers of ice under its dusty surface. Hart's computer-simulated evolution suggests that life on most evolving planets is destroyed by rampant glaciation or suffocation.

The eminent British astronomer Sir Bernard Lovell also favors the anthropic principle. He has determined that the rate of expansion of the universe has to be very precise to permit life. If the universe had expanded a fraction slower than it did, it would have collapsed shortly after its formation. If it had expanded a fraction faster, then gravitationally bound systems like galaxies and solar systems could never have coalesced. Lowell concludes that "chances of the existence of man on earth today, or of intelligent life anywhere in the universe, are vanishingly small."

Pro-ETI and con-ETI forces have already begun to form in the scientific community, and each is drawing heavily on the latest evidence to build its own cogent case. Since the amount of money spent each year on scientific research is very limited, groups on both sides of the ETI issue are sure to engage in heated debate during the coming decades as to how these funds can best be spent. Nevertheless, it is safe to guess that no matter how high the odds rise against the existence of extraterrestrial life, the search will never be abandoned. For we have infinitely more to lose by not exploring the possibility of life on other planets. (See *Our First Close Encounter*, p. 293; and *Listening for Aliens in the 1980s and 1990s*, p. 295.)

Part III

Technology

19

Medical Technology Breakthroughs:
Health Through Computers
and Microelectronics

Computer Diagnosis

By 1990 a computer may serve as your doctor. A computer would flash questions concerning your health on its video screen while you sat at the keyboard terminal and typed in the answers. At the end of the session the computer would type out a complete diagnosis for you — along with its recommendations for medications and treatment. Patients who have been examined by computers claim the impersonal relationship is not in the least objectionable. In fact, they report having been more candid in their responses to very personal questions than they would have been with a doctor.

Carefully designed computer programs, of course, are the key to accurate computer diagnosis. Psychiatrists at the Salt Lake City Veterans' Administration Hospital have been testing one such computer program designed to diagnose mental illnesses. A patient is first greeted by a receptionist, who takes him to a private room and seats him in front of a computer terminal. After the computer completes the formalities of recording the patient's name, address, and social security number, it administers a battery of tests to determine personality factors, I.Q., levels of paranoia and depression, and any suicidal tendencies. This basic computer program includes many branches, or subprograms. If, for example, a patient scores high on the preliminary test for depression, the computer switches to a special depression subprogram to question the patient further on specific aspects of his depression — a feature that not only gives a patient the feeling the computer is listening to him but also that the computer understands his answers. The result of the testing is printed out twenty minutes after the patient has answered the last question, making it possible for a staff psychiatrist to decide quickly whether the patient's problem is serious enough to warrant hospitalization or treatment on an outpatient basis.

Benefits and Accuracy

The Utah psychiatrists have been impressed with the results of their experiment. Computer diagnosis has meant substantial savings in time and money (it costs $500 for a therapist to administer the tests and four days to evaluate them), and patients, too, have benefited from rapid diagnoses. Before the computer testing was initiated, 75 percent of new patients examined by doctors for possible mental problems were hospitalized until their tests were evaluated; with the computer's on-the-spot diagnoses, only 45 percent of the new patients were judged to be in need of constant supervision and were subsequently admitted. Most important, computer diagnosis has proved to be remarkably accurate. In one study involving two groups of institutionalized patients, the computer correctly diagnosed 96 percent of the cases; physicians diagnosed only 83 percent of their patients accurately.

It may seem strange, but the computer was more accurate than the physicians who wrote the computer program. Unlike a human therapist, whose thoroughness of examination, sharpness of perception, and concentration can vary with moods or patient load, the computer's questions are as clear and precisely probing with the day's last patient as they are with the first patient. Also, the computer can never be even unintentionally biased in its evaluation of a patient. And, although it may at first seem ironic, a good deal of the computer's diagnostic edge appears to stem from its impersonal relationship with patients. In one study, 90 percent of the patients claimed they actually preferred revealing their most private problems to a computer, and 56 percent of those patients admitted being more honest with the computer than they would have been with a human therapist.

Computer programs are also being designed to diagnose physical diseases, whose symptoms are usually more clearly defined and evident to the patient himself. Currently, these programs take detailed medical histories, administer psychological tests (to determine if a patient's ailments are largely psychosomatic), then sharply zero in, through a question-and-answer format, on the patient's physical complaints. In a few years the computers are expected to increase greatly their diagnostic accuracy by rapidly analyzing blood, urine, feces, and hair samples obtained from patients by laboratory technicians.

Ultimately, a computer arrives at a diagnosis — and treatment — the same way a doctor does: by matching a patient's symptoms and test results against the wealth of facts known about diseases and cures. Considering a computer's huge, infallible memory, programers claim there is no reason why computers eventually can't be as accurate as physicians in diagnosing disease. Computer diagnosis, of course, is not meant to replace doctors, but to assist them in the quality of services they offer and to allow them to devote more time to those patients who actually require personal attention.

Computer Therapy

It is one thing for a computer to diagnose a patient's mental illness, but it's quite another matter for a computer to play therapist to a patient: "seeing" him twice a week, "listening" to his troubles, and offering advice. Yet scientists are designing computer programs that by the mid 1990s could perform these delicate functions for millions of people.

The leading advocate of computer therapy is Dr. Kenneth Colby, professor of psychiatry at UCLA's Neuropsychiatric Institute and a computer expert. During the 1960s, Dr. Colby attempted to write computer programs that duplicate therapy for specific mental illnesses. Overwhelmed by the complexity of writing programs sufficiently flexible to chart a patient's train of thought and tactfully interrogate him, Colby decided to attack the task in reverse; that is, to write a computer program that simulates the thinking processes of a person suffering from a specific mental problem. He and his colleagues chose paranoia (because its symptoms are among the most well defined of mental disorders), and after a decade of work, they devised PARRY, a program that should make any computer seem paranoid. To test their program, Colby invited a group of psychiatrists to interview a patient, via teletype, who was supposedly in a hospital hundreds of miles away. Each psychiatrist sat at a keyboard and typed questions to the patient, whose answers appeared on a print-out. To Colby's credit, all the psychiatrists diagnosed the patient as paranoid, and not one of them suspected the patient was in reality a computer program.

One advantage of Colby's paranoid "patient" is that it provides psychiatrists with a remarkably credible model of the thought processes of the paranoid mind. By developing programs that simulate other mental illnesses, Colby expects eventually to return to his original goal of writing therapy programs that would enable a computer to treat a patient. After a computer had diagnosed a patient's illness, and that diagnosis was confirmed by a psychiatrist, the computer would select a treatment program. Unlike a psychiatrist who might remain virtually silent during a session, the computer would continually interact with the patient, charting the patient's thought patterns and switching to subprograms whenever necessary to explore particular issues in depth. Eventually the computer's "senses" could be agumented by giving it "ears" and "eyes" so that it could observe a patient. A television camera could inform the computer if, during a particular series of questions, a patient was wringing his or her hands, fidgeting, or pacing the room; a voice analyzer could measure the stress in a patient's responses. Spotting nervousness, stress, or detecting lies, the computer could change its line of questioning to delve deeper into the patient's problem.

No psychiatrist writing computer therapy programs envisions computers treating seriously disturbed patients, but for those thousands of people troubled by mild forms of depression, phobias, and neuroses, a computer could provide the opportunity to abreact. Scientists are divided over the issue of whether computers will ever be sophisticated enough truly to understand a patient's problems, but a cleverly programed computer can appear to understand, sympathize, and even console a troubled patient. Although many psychiatrists and computer experts oppose computer therapy for any person, regardless of how minor the problems, its advocates offer many convincing arguments that they claim are sure to necessitate computer therapy in the next century:

• Cost. Therapists' fees currently range from $45 to $75 an hour and are expected to increase substantially over the next two decades. Thousands of low-to-middle-income people who could benefit from psychiatric therapy but can't afford those rates could afford to "see" a computer several times a week for sessions costing $1.00 an hour.

• Convenience. A session with the indefatigable computer could be scheduled at any hour of the day or night, including Sundays and holidays.

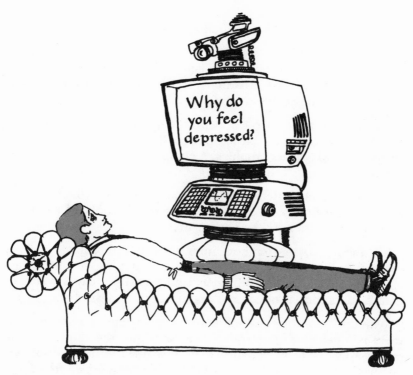

Why do
you feel
depressed?

The Computer as Therapist

Computer programs will treat thousands of people suffering from phobias, neuroses, and depression. An hour session may cost as little as $1.00, and it can be scheduled any time of the day or night and even on Sundays and holidays.

• Fairness. The computer treats all patients objectively.

• Memory. With many patients to treat and a social life outside the office, a psychiatrist may forget facts and feelings confided to her or him; the computer, on the other hand, stores every word and has immediate access to that information. What's more, its recall is always perfect.

• Honesty. Precisely because a computer is nonhuman, a patient may be less embarrassed to confess very human weaknesses and indiscretions that could lie at the foundation of the problems. It is a fact that after many meetings with a psychiatrist, a patient realizes he or she has projected a certain self-image and may attempt either to maintain or to alter that image, at the expense of being perfectly honest.

• Dependability. A psychiatrist gets sick, cancels appointments, and (worst of all) takes vacations. Rain or shine, summer or winter, the computer is always available to "listen."

• Attention. A psychiatrist has problems of his or her own, and there may be times the patient suspects the therapist is more involved with his or her troubles. A computer is always 100 percent attentive.

• Appearance. A patient may feel compelled to be meticulously attired and well groomed when visiting the therapist. A computer couldn't care less how the patient dresses.

• Judgment. No matter how impartial your therapist remains, you may feel he or she passes moral and social judgments on your personal revelations. That fear could easily distort your remarks. A computer, of course, would not think less of you.

• Availability. Advocates of computer therapy point out that there is a dearth of therapists today and that the shortage is expected to worsen. Although it may be argued that it will always be preferable to discuss matters with a concerned therapist, many people may find it's better to "talk" to a computer than to no one at all.

The $12 Million Man

Breakthroughs in the field of bioengineering will soon enable the blind to see, the mute to speak, and the deaf to hear. Many blind and deaf voluunteers are testing prosthetic devices that provide sight and sound through electrodes implanted in the brain's visual center and in the cochlea of the ear. Other prostheses that mimic the functions of body organs will save the lives of cancer and heart-disease patients, and restore to health thousands of people with damaged bladders, blood vessels, testicles, and Fallopian tubes. These are some of the bionic wonders scientists are on the threshold of achieving.

The bionics breakthroughs of the 1980s and 1990s will take advantage of scientists' increasing ability to compress complex computer circuitry that once would have occupied an entire room into a single silicon chip the size of a fingernail. A computer chip programed with instructions on arm movements, for example, makes a bionic arm light and amazingly versatile in the functions it can perform. Stronger and more flexible materials will be responsible for other bionic wonders. Dacron, for instance, currently is used to replace large blood vessels, but because it loses flexibility when stretched into hair-thin tubes, ultrafine Dacron blood vessels are impractical for implantations. Using a new polyurethanelike plastic, however, scientists have constructed ultrafine artifical blood vessels that expand and contract like real vessels when blood pulses through them; and the new plastic, which is being tested in people with severe circulatory problems, appears to be far more durable than Dacron.

Bionics advances are expected to occur at such a breakneck pace over the next two decades that the Armour Engineering Center of the Illinois Institute of Technology has opened an information center in Chicago just to keep doctors abreast of bionics breakthroughs in laboratories around the world.

Electronic Hearing

At present, hearing aids work only if sensory nerves in the ear are still functioning. The lofty goal of researchers, though, is to restore full hearing to the totally deaf. In 1978 British doctors at the University of Melbourne's department of otolaryngology successfully restored partial hearing to a stone-deaf man by implanting ten tiny platinum electrodes in his inner ear. The electrodes were connected to a pea-sized electronic package implanted in the man's mastoid bone, then wound around the man's cochlea. The electrodes never touched the ear's nerve endings, yet they transmitted sounds into the fluid in the cochlea, which in turn stimulated nerves to relay these sound impulses to the brain. The patient, who had lost his hearing in an automobile accident twenty months before the operation, can, with the implant, distinguish sounds of varying pitch and even enjoy music.

Doctors maintain that in order for a patient to achieve full comprehension of speech, at least 100 electrodes would have to be wrapped around the cochlea. This is the goal of the Melbourne researchers for the early 1980s. The recipients of these larger implants must at one time have had the ability to hear to ensure that their brains are programed to interpret sound. Success with these patients will enable doctors to tackle the more complicated problem of providing hearing for children born deaf. With these patients (whose auditory nerves may be completely dead), doctors intend to implant minute electronic sensors in the ears and thread wires directly to the auditory area of the brain, permitting sound waves to by-pass diseased or deadened nerves.

Electronic Vision

Electronic stimulation of the visual centers of the brain is already allowing totally blind patients to "see" silhouettes and distinguish moving and stationary objects. This breakthrough in electronic vision accompanied the discovery in 1968 that blind persons — just like sighted persons — perceive dots of light called phosphenes when the visual cortex at the back of the brain is stimulated with an electric current. Researchers realized that if a sufficient number of electrodes were implanted in the visual cortex, they could draw images with the dots that would enable the blind person to "see."

In 1975 a team of Utah surgeons separated the two brain hemispheres of a man who had been blinded in a gunshot accident. Against the visual section of his brain they rested a two-inch-square Teflon wafer studded with sixty-four electrodes, and then allowed the brain halves to come together again gently, holding the wafer in place. Wires led from the electrodes to a nickel-sized opening in the patient's skull just behind his right ear, converging to form a plug-in socket. When the doctors connected the wires to a computer, which was in turn connected to a television camera aimed at a horizontal strip of white tape on a dark background, the patient saw a horizontal line of forty-two bright phosphene dots (the electrode-phosphene ratio is not one-to-one). Since then he has learned to use dot images to distinguish geometric shapes and to read Braille sentences much faster than he can with his fingers.

Dr. William Dobelle of New York's Columbia Presbyterian Medical Center is continuing work with this patient in order further to improve his vision, and asserts that phosphene images can be greatly enhanced for him and other blind people. Dr. Dobelle expected to experiment with larger implants, ranging from 256 to 512 electrodes, on other patients during the 1980s. Eventually he plans to miniaturize the electronics so that a blind person, surgically equipped with 1024 electrodes, could see with the aid of a tiny television camera mounted on frames of dummy eyeglasses. The camera would serve as the person's eyes, surveying the environment, while the electrodes created dot pictures as legible as those you see on electronic scoreboards in sports stadiums. In time, researchers claim, they should be able to implant television cameras the size of hazel nuts directly into the eye sockets, and conceal the rest of the system's electronics in the stems of spectacles.

Electronic Speech

As long as a mute person possesses vocal muscles, he may be able to talk even though his vocal cords may have been damaged or surgically removed. Researchers are developing ultrasensitive electrodes to be implanted in throat muscles and connected to a small computer and speaker that a person would wear in his shirt pocket. The electrodes would detect the speaker's pre-word electrical impulses (or vibrations) and relay these impulses to the computer, which would convert them into human-sounding speech. This system of electronic speech is more difficult to develop than either electronic hearing or vision; it requires a knowledge of words in their pre-spoken electrical impulses, as well as a computer that can convincingly mimic the human voice over a range of vocabulary large enough to make electronic speech both practical and desirable. Bionics engineers claim realistic electronic speech is possible and that the first system could be tested with mute persons by the end of the century.

The Bionic Arm and Hand

Scientists at the University of Utah's Projects and Design Laboratory are perfecting an artificial arm and hand that picks up electrical signals from muscles in an amputee's stump, shoulder, upper back, and chest. Electrodes relay these impulses to a tiny powerpack strapped to the body that transmits them to miniatuure motors in the mechanical arm and hand. Since these electricial impulses contain all the information necessary to move a real arm, by cleverly designed electronics the impulses can be used to make the movements of an artificial arm astonishingly real.

At its present stage of development the two-pound, $3000 myoelectric arm bends at the elbow and rotates at the wrist, and its hand opens, closes, and can lift a weight of about three pounds — more than enough strength to perform most daily activities. According to volunteers fitted with the myoelectric arm, they need only think of a motion to perform it. The muscle-operated hand is being improved to include additional finger movements that will provide nearly as much dexterity as a real hand. A myoelectric

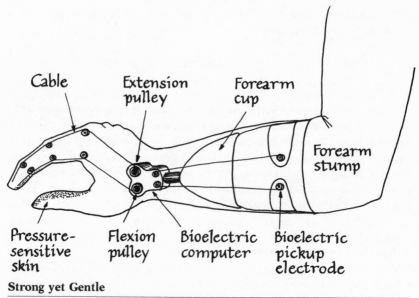

Cable   Extension   Forearm
         pulley   cup

Forearm
stump

Pressure-   Flexion   Bioelectric   Bioelectric
sensitive   pulley   computer   pickup
skin   electrode

Strong yet Gentle

Operated by electrical muscle impulses from a person's upper arm or shoulder, the ultimate artificial arm will possess wrist and finger movements of astonishing dexterity. Pressure-sensitive electronic skin will make the hand feel almost real to the user.

leg that operates on the same principle of electrical impulses is also being designed.

Electronic Touch

One requirement of the ideal bionic hand is that it be strong enough to lift a frying pan yet gentle enough to grip a crystal goblet without crushing it. This variable strength may come from the development of electronic touch. Scientists are designing thin, electronically sensitized plastic to serve as skin over the fingers and palms of bionic hands. Simulating the behavior of nerves, fine sensors in the plastic skin would detect pressure and instantaneously relay impulses to the user, enabling him to control the power of his grip. When perfected, the sensors will function so sensitively that a person wearing a bionic hand may actually feel that he has regained his sense of touch. In time, his artificial hand may seem real. Ultimately, bionics engineers expect to be able to cover artificial feet with similar electric skin to assure a person with an artificial leg firm footing.

Electronic Spinal Cord

In many paralyzed patients nerves in one or more vertebrae are damaged to the extent that they cannot relay signals to the brain. If these broken circuits along the spinal cord could be repaired, the patient could regain movement. Doctors at the Veterans' Administration Hospital in Maryland are working on electrical bridges that would span damaged vertebrae, thus shunting vital signals past the dead nerves. The bridges consist of webs of fine wires that simulate the ability of nerves to transmit electric current. If these spinal-cord bridges perform as well as doctors anticipate, by 1990 thousands of people now regarded as paralytics may recover enough movement to leave their sickbeds and wheelchairs and become self-reliant.

. . .

Electronic or mechanical equivalents to virtually every major organ in the body are on the drawing boards of engineers. Increasing the durability of these prostheses, powering them with safe, long-lived batteries, and connecting them to minicomputers that will regulate functions, constitute the goals of bionics research. The key that has opened the bionics era, of course, is computer miniaturization. Scientists foresee the day when a computer, containing all the words in a dictionary or information in an encyclopedia, could be small enough to fit inside a tooth and wired to our brain. If you were stumped on the spelling or definition of a word, forgot the date of Verdi's death or the dawn of Minoan civilization, all you would have to do is query the memory in your tooth for the answers. The possibility of lifelike bionic arms and legs, electronic eyes and ears, sensitive artificial skin, and the knowledge of the world stored in a tooth makes the development of a completely bionic person — the perfect robot — an almost unbelievable, yet probable, reality.

Supermagnetic Medicine

A physicist's tool known as nuclear magnetic resonance (NMR) may in a decade become every physician's diagnostic dream. NMR could inform your doctor what's occurring at the very core of your body's cells, and be used to destroy diseased or genetically defective cells — all without damaging healthy tissues.

To appreciate the tremendous potential of NMR you must understand how the technique provides a window into the heart of a cell. The nuclei of almost all atoms can act as tiny magnets. In the presence of an externally applied magnetic field, these magnets wobble at their own particular frequencies. If you beam radio-frequency (RF) signals at the wobbling nuclei, they'll absorb that energy and resonate. When the RF field is shut off, the nuclei emit the energy they've absorbed as their own characteristic signature, a sort of fingerprint of the state of fitness of an atom or molecule. For over thirty years physicists have been identifying the magnetic signatures of molecules, and now medical researchers are ready to work with these signatures in diagnosing diseases.

At the University of Pennsylvania School of Medicine doctors are attempting to perfect a technique that would permit them to take an NMR picture of a heart patient's chest to determine the actual number of cells that were destroyed during the heart attack. They've already determined that dead or damaged heart cells have particular magnetic signatures. Once refined, the technique could be used to measure the amount of damage to brain cells from a stroke. (This breakthrough may occur sooner than the Pennsylvania researchers imagine. In early 1979, scientists at the British electronics company EMI succeeded in taking the world's first magnetic pictures of a cross-section of a patient's brain, an achievement that's bound to accelerate NMR research.) Scientists at the University of Illinois Medical Center are recording NMR traces of healthy and dystrophic muscles to locate the biochemical cause of muscular dystrophy. Because NMR yields information directly from the center of cells, researchers feel the technique has almost limitless potential. At the University of Oxford in England, doctors are developing a technique to assess the cellular state of health of an organ before it's transplanted into a patient. A breakthrough in this area could greatly increase the success of transplants, especially of kidneys, since recent studies have shown that most transplanted kidneys fail not because the recipient's immune system rejects them, but because the organs were marred by deep-rooted cellular damage that had escaped the most discerning doctor's eye.

Shooting Cancer Cells

Though most of these techniques are at least a decade away, one physician has already begun to use NMR on an experimental basis to search for early signs of cancer. At the Downstate Medical Center in Brooklyn, New York, Dr. Raymond Damadian has constructed an enormous supermagnet. If you sit snugly within its skein of coils, the very atoms in your body begin to wobble. You're then shot with a radio-frequency beam. It's a perfectly harmless experience; you don't feel even a tingle. Dr. Damadian has shown that NMR can detect subtle differences between healthy and tumorous tissues: cancer cells are slower to release the RF signals they've absorbed. Working with women, Damadian has learned that breast tumors and cancerous lung tissue give back their RF signals at different times. He believes that in the future pathologists will depend on NMR to understand the exact chemistry of various diseased cells. "With NMR the body's own natural elements can be made to broadcast their own state of health or disease," says Damadian. "The beauty of NMR is that it's non-invasive. You don't need surgery or X-rays. The RF signals are like the radio and TV signals we're constantly exposed to."

Where diagnosis with NMR may occur in the late 1980s, the treatment of disease through nuclear magnetic resonance may lie an additional ten years in the future. Damadian, whose research is perhaps the furthest advanced of anyone's today, likes to speculate on the therapeutic applications of NMR. "We might be able to beam in destructive radio signals at a cancerous tissue alone. Healthy cells would be unharmed since they wouldn't absorb energy at that frequency." He's currently testing that possibility, along with mapping the signatures of various cancers. Once the magnetic signatures of diseases are identified and catalogued, NMR could grow into a significant diagnostic tool.

Diagnosing with Magnetic Fields

You're familiar with the diagnostic powers of the EEG and the ECG that trace brainwave rhythms and heartbeat patterns. But what about the MEG and the MCG? The MEG monitors your brain and the MCG your heart, but unlike the electroencephalograph and electrocardiograph, which measure electric currents, the magnetoencephalograph (MEG) and the magnetocardiograph (MCG) describe the much subtler magnetic fields that emanate from your brain and heart. Within a decade doctors will be taking magnetic readings of your heart and brain and diagnosing ailments that they would have missed with conventional electric-current traces.

Preliminary work with MCGs shows they reveal abnormalities in strength of the heart muscle and nonuniformity of its beat that the conventional ECG could never detect; in this way they may prove to be the earliest warning system of heart trouble. As for the MEG, magnetic traces of the brains of sleeping persons are revealing new stages in the pattern of sleep so thoroughly different from the familiar ones traced by the EEG that scientists still aren't sure how to interpret the information. Even at this early stage, MEG research is making it clear that sleep (and probably many other brain functions, especially memory and recall) is more complex than scientists have estimated.

At New York University, Dr. Samuel Williamson has used magnetic readings to study peoples' response times. In one experiment young men and women were shown complex patterns and asked to press a button to signal when they had fully grasped a particular pattern. Williamson was not surprised to learn that the more complicated a pattern, the longer a person's response time, yet the magnetograms led to a startling discovery: the various reaction times did not correlate with how fast a pattern was visually perceived. In fact, the visual cortex of the brain in all the volunteers seemed to comprehend a pattern in the same amount of time; the different rates of pushing the button were due to the volunteers' particular motor responses. Some merely moved slower than others. For an unknown reason, their network of nerves may relay commands from the brain at a more sluggish pace. Williamson predicts that magnetograms will eventually create new fields in the psychology and physiology of human behavior.

One advantage of the MCG and MEG is that they can be administered without skin contact. This means they are faster and easier than the ECG and EEG, and the electric potential of a person's skin doesn't blur the reading, as happens when contact electrodes are used. Another advantage of the MCG is that it can sense the effects of direct heart current (DC), but the ECG can detect only the effects of alternating current (AC), thus missing an entire behavior pattern of the heart. What's responsible for the development of MEGs and MCGs is a new, exquisitely sensitive magnetic detector called a SQUID (Superconducting Quantum Interference Device). SQUIDs are capable of detecting a magnetic field one-billionth the strength of the earth's magnetic field, and just about the level of the body's magnetism.

Mental Magnetism

By 1985 you should know the results of at least two fascinating studies now underway. In one, MEGs are being taken of both severe psychotic patients and normal people. Even the psychiatrists performing the study can't estimate the variety of brainwave patterns or the practical applications of their research. In a broader study, MCGs are being recorded for people with healthy hearts as well as patients suffering from just about every kind of heart ailment known. The MCGs will then be studied by experienced cardiologists to establish norms and criteria for distinguishing healthy from diseased hearts. An MCG and an ECG of your heart should enable your doctor to diagnose — and perhaps predict the probability of — heart problems with a high degree of accuracy. Some researchers believe that magnetograms may also turn out to be acutely sensitive detectors of tumors in their earliest stage of growth.

Magnetoencephalograms may also prove a boon to the field of altered states of consciousness research. The EEG reveals that the brainwaves of a hypnotized subject are identical to those of a person fully awake, a fact that has perplexed some researchers and prompted others to claim that there is nothing unique about a trance. An MEG, on the other hand, may be capable of differentiating between a wakeful and a mesmerized mind, a difference that psychologists hope can be measured objectively. MEGs may also elucidate subtle differences between the mind of a person meditating or engaged in creative cognition. EEGs show that alpha brainwaves (twelve to eight cycles per second) and theta brainwaves (seven to three cycles per second) are rough indicators of these activities; MEGs may hone the differences even more finely. Over the decade of the 1980s, we'll see magnetic traces progress from the hottest experimental toy of researchers to powerful medical tools that will save lives and provide fresh insights into our bodies and minds.

Transparent Bodies

Since the discovery of X rays, doctors have succeeded in peering ever more closely at the human body. By the late 1980s, with the perfection of a sophisticated radiological technique, positron emission tomography (PET), they will be able to examine the body with unimaginable clarity. Using PET, radiologists can observe minute anatomical details, and for the first time photograph body chemistry in progress — whether it's an emphysema victim's red blood cells struggling to draw oxygen from lung tissue, or portions of the brain being activated as a person speaks or reads. With PET, it will be possible for the doctor to follow on a video screen the action of drugs in the body at a cellular level and thus intimately monitor recovery from disease. In fact, PET scanners promise to reveal so many of our body's internal processes that the scanners should greatly reduce the need for biopsies and dangerous exploratory surgery. To appreciate PET fully, it is necessary to understand the related breakthrough — CAT (computer axial tomography).

CAT Scanners

Currently, there are two nonsurgical means of investigating the body: through the external application of X rays, or by injecting radioactively tagged chemicals into the body and tracing their emissions. CAT scanners operate on this first procedure; PET scanners on the second. Like all X-ray devices, a CAT scanner fires a measured amount of radiation into the body and, by detecting the residue that emerges, creates pictures of body organs. CAT scanners, perfected in the late 1970s, are more impressive than mere X-ray machines — they're technological marvels.

A CAT scanner consists of an X-ray tube and detector that are mounted on opposite sides of a patient; they rotate around the patient's body, snapping scores of X-ray pictures in a matter of minutes. A computer processes these individual snapshots and then creates on a video screen a cross-sectional view of the patient's body — as though the body had been cleanly sliced and photographed perpendicular to the cut. A visual slice can be taken through any portion of the body, and many closely spaced slices can be combined to form the complete picture of an organ. With this information stored in a computer, a doctor can choose to display a view of an organ from any perspective, slice an organ through any plane, or activate a zoom lens for close-up examination of particular features. In fact, for a doctor, a CAT image of an organ is the next best thing to holding the organ in his hand.

CAT scanners have just begun to allow radiologists to follow the spread of sclerosis through the liver, and the crawl of cancer within one organ and as it metastasizes to other organs. CAT's full potential for diagnosing disease will be explored during the 1980s.

Despite their tremendous versatility, however, CAT scanners (which cost up to $2 million) have one disadvantage: like all X-ray devices, their image represents a mixture of radiation from different depths of the body compressed onto the flat plane of a film. Thus, regions of high radiation intensity (hot spots) can mask less intense areas behind or in front of them. Vital details can be lost. This is not the case with the more versatile PET scanners.

PET Scanners

A PET scanner detects radiation emitted from a patient's body after he has swallowed, inhaled, or been injected with a drug tagged with a radioactive element. To avoid photographing, and superimposing, this radiation from different depths in the body, a PET scanner's camera continuously changes focus as it sweeps over a patient. Each different focus records information from one specific depth so that no region obscures another. From these thousands of individual pictures a computer constructs a cross-sectional image of the body.

With PET scanners, the body's exposure to radiation is minimized because the drugs are tagged with radioactive elements that shed most of their radiation quickly — within several minutes to a few hours — through the emission of subatomic particles called positrons. Since drugs tagged with positrons must be freshly prepared shortly before they are administered to a patient, scientists working with PET scanners must have ready access to high-energy accelerators. To date, researchers have tagged numerous drugs, as well as alcohol, sugar, amino acids, fats, and proteins, with positrons.

Even at this early stage of research, PET scanners are dazzling doctors with new images of the body. At the Brookhaven National Laboratory, one of six centers in the United States conducting PET studies, radiologists injected radioactively tagged glucose (sugar water) into a patient and then scanned his brain while he raised and lowered his right arm. The PET images revealed a positron hot spot on the left side of the brain in the precise region that controls right-arm movements; the man's mental activity was causing that part of his brain to metabolize glucose faster than in the rest of the brain. When other subjects have been injected with tagged glucose and then had their right hands stroked by doctors, the PET scans revealed increases in glucose metabolism in their brains' sensory and motor areas corresponding to that hand.

Scientists are also using PET scanners to probe the brain's visual and auditory centers. In one experiment a patient injected with tagged glucose had his right eye covered with a patch while he studied different geometrical shapes with his left eye. PET pictures of his brain revealed quiescence in his left brain hemisphere (which registers right-eye perception), and several spots of vigorous activity in his right hemisphere. The activity reflected — in ways scientists have yet fully to comprehend — the brain's processing of visual information. At the University of Pennsylvania scientists conducted experiments in which people listened to a story while one ear was covered with a soundproof muff. The researchers were astonished to observe that regardless of which ear was left uncovered, the greatest brain activity always occurred in the more creatively oriented right hemisphere. The scientists think they have isolated an area in the right hemisphere that collates a multitude of facts into a coherent story. Eventually researchers intend to test children with learning disabilities to determine how different areas of their brain perceive, store, and correlate sounds and images. In this way neurologists may be able to pinpoint areas of low metabolic activity that could be responsible for a child's inability to learn.

Drug Activity

PET scanners also create images of cells. Doctors at the Hôpital d'Orsay in France are using their scanner to locate damaged cells in the brains of stroke victims and to monitor — at a cellular level — the patients' road to recovery. In related research in the United States, scientists have relied on PET scanners to study the damaged hearts of heart-attack patients, and have been able to see destroyed muscle tissue. Such insights could eventually suggest new treatments for stroke and heart-attack victims.

The PET scanner at the University of California at Los Angeles is being used to study the brain activity of epileptics. Researchers there have located specific areas of the brain where metabolism and blood flow are abnormally low and where they become abnormally high during a seizure. Other scientists have identified reduced metabolism in the brains of schizophrenics, and are just beginning to determine why antipsychotic drugs are more effective with some patients than others. Eventually, PET images of the stomach and intestines of obese people fed radioactively tagged fats could reveal how and why they metabolize these fats less efficiently than thin people.

The potential of PET scanners to map brain activity, chart the effects of drug action, and follow the spread or remission of disease at a cellular level has prompted the National Institutes of Health to grant $10 million for further research. Although PET technology already exists, doctors are seeking to perfect the medical procedures that could elevate PET scanners into the medical marvels of the 1990s. In making the body transparent, PET scanners will greatly increase our understanding of disease and dramatically reduce the need for many kinds of surgery.

Seeing with Sound

Obstetricians have depended on high-frequency sound waves — ultrasonography — since the early 1960s to examine fetuses for abnormalities. Ultrasonography poses no radiation threat and can detect features ten times smaller than those shown by X ray, and ultrasound devices are cheaper to buy and operate than X-ray equipment. By the mid 1980s, newer ultrasound machines are expected to acquire a degree of sophistication that promises to revolutionize the field of ultrasound medicine. One eagerly anticipated breakthrough is the possibility of producing ultrasound "signatures" of healthy and diseased tissues, thus enabling doctors to distinguish malignant from benign tumors, eliminating the need for biopsies.

The principle behind ultrasonography is amazingly simple. Sound frequencies up to five million cycles per second — well beyond the range that can be heard by the most sensitive animal ears — are bounced off a fetus (or body organ) to create echoes. As a speaker captures the echoes, a computer translates them into pictures of the object deflecting the sound. Bouncing sound off a fetus floating in amniotic fluid is like using sonar to detect details of the ocean floor. In fact, ultrasonography is a technological spin-off of sonar. Existing ultrasound devices are sensitive enough to capture the features of a baby's profile in the thirteenth week of pregnancy, the baby's internal organs in the twentieth week, and the genitals in the third trimester, providing absolute sex determination. Even more astonishing feats will be possible with the new ultrasound equipment that is expected to be readily available in this decade.

Doppler Diagnosis

Just as Doppler radar bounces sound off a car to measure the car's speed, a Doppler ultrasonograph will allow doctors to measure the rate of blood flow through a fetus's heart as early as the eighth week after conception. Early knowledge of a fetus's heart activity can mean the difference between a healthy delivery and a stillbirth or a spontaneous abortion. A slow heartbeat, for instance, may indicate that the baby's constitution is especially weak and that the mother should assume a more relaxed life style, give up alcohol and cigarettes, and fortify her body through better nutrition.

These ultrasonographs also will be capable of finer resolution of detail, a fact that could spell the difference between life or death in certain kinds of pregnancy. For instance, in an ectopic pregnancy — one in which the fetus is not developing in the uterus but usually in one of the Fallopian tubes — doctors will be able to spot the displaced fetus earlier than is now possible and surgically correct the problem before the fetus grows so large that it ruptures the tube, causing the mother a possibly fatal hemorrhage.

Men, too, stand to benefit from sharper ultrasound techniques. Within a few years ultrasound specialists expect to be able to make images of cross-sections of the coronary arteries feeding the heart. In this way ultrasound could provide a harmless, nonintrusive procedure for detecting telltale signs of atherosclerosis and directly measuring how badly arteries are clogged.

Sound Movies

In the past, only still pictures could be taken with sound waves, but a device, a real-time scanner, is changing that. By sweeping over an object that's in the process of reflecting sound waves, a real-time scanner produces motion pictures. This device is so sensitive it detects the movements of a fetus as early as six weeks after conception — well before a mother can feel her baby move. With a real-time scanner, the obstetrician will be able to observe the fetus as it shifts position, sucks its thumb — and breathes. Of course, a fetus does not breathe air, but throughout gestation a baby's chest rises and falls in motions resembling normal breathing. Doctors are puzzled by this action and unsure of its significance; they believe that the real-time scanner is the first device that will allow them to unravel the meaning of this mysterious motion.

Mongolism

Within a few short years, improved techniques of examining ultrasonograms should make it possible to detect certain genetic defects early in pregnancy in time for a safe abortion. According to British doctors at the Clinical Research Center at London's

Northwick Park Hospital, the first genetic disease to be reliably diagnosed from the ultrasonogram will most likely be Down's syndrome, or mongolism. A fetus with Down's syndrome possesses an extra chromosome that results in widely spaced eyes and an abnormally flat pelvis. At present the condition is diagnosed by the technique of amniocentesis in which fetal cells are extracted from the amniotic fluid with a needle and subjected to a chromosome test. The abnormal features of a mongoloid fetus, however, can be only faintly detected in the fifteenth week of pregnancy with present ultrasound techniques. The London doctors assert that in the near future ultrasonograms could be used for much earlier diagnosis of mongolism. (Since the physical shape of a baby even after birth is not uncontestable evidence of Down's syndrome, a chromosome test by amniocentesis would still be needed to confirm beyond doubt the ultrasound diagnosis.)

British researchers are also developing ultrasound techniques to measure the shape and size of a fetus's liver to determine if the fetus is suffering from malnutrition, in which case the mother's diet would be improved. The doctors are also using sound to obtain an image of the partition between the pumping chambers of a fetus's heart. A rupture in the partition interferes with blood circulation, producing "blue babies." As long as the baby is in the womb receiving oxygen from its mother's blood, the rupture does not present a hazard, but after birth the defect immediately begins to threaten the child's life. In a few years ultrasound techniques could be used to diagnose a blue baby before birth, enabling doctors to make arrangements for surgically mending the hole immediately after birth. Because of the anticipated advances in ultrasonography and the safety of the procedure, ultrasound examinations may become routine for pregnant women by the mid-to-late 1980s.

Hidden Worlds

The conventional microscope focuses with light waves to create images of cells and their components. But microscopes that create images using sound waves promise to be even more powerful tools for probing the interior world of cells. By the end of the decade, acoustic microscopes may afford doctors early and accurate diagnoses of diseases at a cellular level, and supply the first pictures revealing how nerves relay commands throughout the body.

The tremendous diagnostic potential of sound microscopes has been known for three decades, but only within the last few years have scientists mastered the technology required for constructing acoustic microscopes. Researchers at Stanford University have designed an acoustic microscope that produces a narrowly focused beam of sound waves vibrating at three billion cycles per second. Sound waves this small can probe the features of a micro-organism with the same accuracy as light waves. Whereas light bounces off a micro-organism and relays information about its surface details, the tiny sound waves actually penetrate the surface to reveal internal features.

Tests with acoustic microscopes indicate that they can measure important biological properties of cells, particularly a cell's elasticity. Cancer cells and sickle cells, for example, have abnormal elasticities that, under an acoustic microscope, show up as differences in the velocity of sound waves through the cells. The increased elasticity of cancer cells is considered to be the property that permits them to metastasize throughout the body by slipping through narrow passages that block the migration of normal cells. By measuring the elasticity of a sample of cells from a patient's tumor, doctors could determine the probability of the tumor's spreading to various parts of the body.

Two types of acoustic microscopes are being tested: the scanning acoustic microscope (SAM), and the scanning laser acoustic microscope (SLAM). The major difference between SAM and SLAM is that the latter does not focus sound waves onto a specific point of the object under investigation. Instead, SLAM spreads its sound waves uniformly over the surface of the sample organism. The reflected sound waves form an image whose vibrations are scanned by a laser and interpreted as a picture. This process is analogous to the espionage technique in which a laser beam is focused on a window to detect conversations on the opposite side of the glass by measuring how the sound waves vibrate the glass.

Scientists are just beginning to mine the many possible functions of acoustic microscopes. Dr. Reginald C. Eggleton of the Indiana University Medical School, for one, is studying the effects of drugs on individual heart cells, as well as tracing the pathway of nerve impulses that travel out from the heart when it is stimulated by a pacemaker. These cells don't have to be stained (as with an optical microscope) or exposed to a dehydrating vacuum (as is necessary with an electron microscope) to be seen, but can be viewed in their natural state — an advantage of the acoustic microscope that has elated biologists. Also, many industries expect to work with acoustic microscopes to search for defects in integrated chips (a basic part of computers and various electronic devices), ceramics, semiconductors, and for dangerous stresses in metals. The ability of acoustic microscopes to penetrate objects — without the hazards of X-rays — offers industry a safe technique for analyzing materials and saving millions of dollars. The contribution to us could be invaluable.

20

Communications Breakthroughs:
Toward a Smaller, More Convenient World

Living by Phone

Short dialing, call announcing, and call monitoring represent a few of the features that will revolutionize telephone communications in the 1980s. Emphasizing speed and the caller's convenience, scientists are wedding microelectronics and minicomputers to develop the next generation of phones for our homes, offices, and cars. Today's copper-cable telephone lines will be replaced by hair-thin glass fibers capable of carrying vast amounts of information on pulses of laser light. Fiber telephone lines could transform the picture phone into a commonplace reality. By connecting the phones of the future to versatile home computers, you will be able to shop, pay bills, and read library books from a typewriter keyboard and television screen in your living room.

Several of the simpler phone features are already available in various parts of the country. By the end of the decade they could provide standard services in every household.

Short Dialing

This is a feature you're sure to appreciate if you're busy or impatient. Future phones will contain a built-in memory for frequently called numbers. Instead of dialing or pushing the buttons for all the digits of a particular number, you need push only the first two or three digits. The phone's memory will instantly recognize the number and immediately complete your call.

Call Forwarding

If you're usually on the move you will particularly be interested in this feature, which will automatically allow you to receive calls miles away from your home or office. All that's necessary is to punch the number of the phone where you can be reached on your home or business phone. A phone company computer will then forward any incoming calls to the number you've designated.

Call Announcing

This feature will be especially helpful in emergencies or urgent situations when you must reach someone who happens to be using the phone. By simply pressing a "beep" button, you'll be able to signal that person you are trying to get through to, without having the operator interrupt the conversation. The person you're calling can then beep you back to acknowledge that he's aware of your incoming call. Of course, the system will allow people to develop special beep codes within families and among friends and business associates to establish just who is calling. For instance, one long and two short incoming beeps might indicate that your spouse is trying to get through; your answer, three short beeps, could indicate that your call can't be interrupted and you'll return his or her call as soon as possible.

Call Monitoring

This service offers just the solution for people who hate to redial. With call monitoring you can dial a number and if it's busy you won't have to dial it again. Your phone will automatically monitor the desired number and complete the call as soon as that line becomes free.

Call Shunting

This feature can be used to give the polite brush-off as well as to protect your privacy. Is there someone you don't care to talk with? Dial his number, push a special shunt button, and every time he calls you from that number he'll get a busy signal. If you suspect he may also try calling later in the day from another phone, you can shunt that number, too. Call shunting could, however, be rendered obsolete by the 1990s. By that time, a feature called "number display" will flash the number of an incoming caller on a small panel on your phone. Recognizing the number, you would then have the option to answer or not.

• • •

Future phones will not only be more fun to use, but service will be faster and more reliable because of two upcoming innovations:

Computer Operators

A computerized voice rather than a human voice will soon be answering directory-assistance requests. Once you've spelled the name of the person whose number you want, the computer will locate it automatically. If you also provide the person's street address, the computer will thank you for the extra information and reward you by finding the number faster. Even your misspelling a name (within reason) will not confuse the computer.

Will computers ultimately be capable of identifying people by their voices and thus serve as security systems? Scientists are learning that, though it's relatively easy to program a computer to "talk" — and even to "understand" spoken numbers, letters, and words — it's incredibly more difficult to perfect a computer voice-recognition system. Whereas a talking computer is programed with either taped human speech or sounds and syllables from which it constructs its own words, a voice-recognition computer must be able to distinguish the tens of thousands of subtle differences in pitch, inflection, rhythm, and dialect that characterize voices. Voices may be as distinctive as fingerprints, but scientists claim that the perfect voice-recognition computer that will permit you to transfer money from bank accounts to stores without the danger of an impersonator dipping into your funds is about twenty years in the future.

Light Conversation

Telephone cables made of thin threads of ultrapure glass will permit many more calls to be transmitted at the same time — interference free — over beams of laser light. This system, fiber optics communications, is based on pulses of light generated by a miniature laser to carry voice, data, and video signals through transparent fibers the thickness of human hair. Light signals in optical fibers can convey much more information than electrical signals in conventional copper cables. For instance, a bundle of twenty fibers no thicker than a pencil can handle 76,200 calls daily. By comparison, a copper cable three inches in diameter and containing 1800 individual wires transports only 900 conversations. The flexible fiber bundles have several additional features that enhance their appeal: they weigh only 1 percent as much as copper cables (which makes them easier to lay and repair); they occupy far less space under city streets and pavements; and, since they are composed of pure glass, they will never corrode. Furthermore, electrical signals in copper wire need to be reamplified by special boosters every 300 to 6000 feet, but the same signals can run for many miles in optical fibers without the necessity of reamplification.

Fiber optics systems have been successfully tested by American Telephone and Telegraph in Chicago, and by General Telephone and Electronics in Santa Monica, California. Bell Telephone scientists plan to begin replacing copper cables with fiber bundles in high-density call areas in the mid-to-late 1980s. Eventually the entire country will be laced with these marvelous fibers, making phone service more reliable and versatile. "Tomorrow's telephone will become the key to a broad communications and information center," predicts AT&T chairman Charles Brown. "People will be able to call up data storage banks, libraries, newspapers and magazines to request and automatically receive pictures and printed information about news events, fashion, sports, travel, books — almost any subject. They may use their phones to vote in elections, to bank by credit cards, to make and charge purchases from department stores or to play bridge coast to coast using video monitors."

A Ring of Satellites

As optical fibers promise to revolutionize communications between cities and states, orbiting "geosynchronous" satellites should revolutionize global communications. Geosynchronous satellites circle the earth once a day 22,400 miles above the equator, and thus they remain fixed over one geographical location. At the end of 1978 twenty such communications satellites were in orbit, transmitting live news, sports events, and entertainment to millions of people throughout the world. By 1990, dozens more geosynchronous satellites are expected to ring the earth in a silvery necklace. This satellite network will provide an instant worldwide telecasting capacity of 22,000 television channels, enabling viewers in, for example, Montclair, New Jersey, to watch live local news coverage in Florence, Italy.

Many of the communications satellites will be owned by private companies and used by businesses and individuals. Companies will rely on these satellites to hold "electronic conferences." A Georgia-based company recently staged a three-hour sales meeting via satellite: television screens, microphones, and loud speakers enabled the company's 2000 employees in eleven different cities to watch, and fully participate in, the meeting, which originated at the company's Atlanta headquarters. Had the company flown their employees to the meeting, the tab would have amounted to $600,000; the electronic conference cost half that amount.

These more economical conferences will surely become increasingly popular — and even less expensive — when the space shuttle begins to fly. The shuttle will be used to put into orbit new communications satellites and retrieve them inexpensively for repair, thus indefinitely extending a satellite's present seven-year life span and making it more economical to use.

In fact, satellite communication is expected to boom over the next few years. Revenue from commercial satellites totaled $420 million at the end of 1978, and it is estimated to reach $1 billion by 1983. Experts predict that communications satellites eventually will carry the bulk of world communications and that developing nations will sidestep the usual stage of long-distance ground systems and depend solely on satellites. By the end of this century, it may even be possible for people on different sides of the globe to take advantage of geosynchronous satellites to communicate by small wrist radios.

The Truth Box

Telephones soon may be turned into miniature lie detectors by being equipped with tiny electronic devices that could measure emotional stress in a caller's voice and suggest if a person is avoiding the truth. Even smaller versions of the voice lie detector will be built into digital watches. Although the phone and watch "truth boxes" are likely to discourage prevarication, they threaten to invade our privacy and may open a Pandora's box of ethical and legal problems.

These truth-checking devices are miniaturized versions of the Psychological Stress Evaluator (PSE) now commonplace with police departments, the FBI, and the CIA. Though the conventional lie detector, or polygraph, records changes in blood pressure, breathing, and the skin's electrical conductivity — responses that indicate lying — the PSE picks up modulations, or "microtremors," in a person's voice. These microtremors — too slight to be detected by our ears — vary according to the degree of stress. The PSE, in its present state of technology, is less accurate at detecting lies than the conventional polygraph, but refinements are expected over the next few years.

One mini–PSE for home or office use is already available, though psychologists debate its accuracy. It's the size of a cigarette carton, weighs two pounds, and can be easily attached to a telephone. This mini–PSE measures the caller's voice for low stress on a row of one to eight green lights, and high stress on a row of red lights. The machine includes a built-in recorder that can tape a conversation and play it back later so that the caller's veracity can be double-checked.

Unlike polygraphs, which have to be wired to a person's body, a PSE has only to record a person's voice to determine if he or she is lying. Thus, PSEs lend themselves to an almost limitless variety of covert uses, from an employer concealing a mini–PSE in the desk drawer as he interviews a prospective employee, to a teacher wearing a mini–detector watch as he questions a student about cheating on a test. Such use of PSEs is frightening, particularly when we consider that the person interrogated may well be telling the truth, but because of the stressfulness of the situation — or, more likely, the inability of the unprofessional interrogator accurately to interpret a PSE's output — may be accused of lying. These Big Brother implications of PSEs have so concerned the federal government that it is considering legislation to regulate strictly the sale and use of voice lie detectors.

The first versions of the miniaturized voice lie detectors are expected in 1980. However, many lie detector experts challenge the accuracy of these devices and their reliability in the hands of untrained persons. "You could read anything you want into the flashing lights," says one expert. "For an amateur, the mini–PSEs will be about as accurate a barometer of behavior as a mood ring." More sophisticated and reliable versions of these small voice lie detectors will likely appear in the late 1980s. By the time this occurs, a license to own a PSE may be required, and under the penalty of law you may have to warn people when your PSE is recording their voices.

Car Phones for All

By 1990 every car driver may have a phone in his or her car. These car phones will be far more sophisticated than CB radios. In fact, car phones eventually will serve as extensions of the future home phones and, as such, be as versatile.

To date, the use of car and hand-held phones has been limited because of an insufficient number of radio frequencies. The "grid cell," however — already approved by the Federal Communications Commission — offers an ingenious solution to this problem. Current car phone systems depend on a single transmitter and receiver to service all phones in a geographical area. Thus, a particular radio frequency is available to only one phone in that area at a time. Under the grid-cell system, cities will be partitioned into areas, or cells, each covering a few square miles. Every area will then be assigned its own transmitting and receiving computer, allowing for many more calls on each frequency band. In this way, dozens of drivers in several different areas of each city can broadcast over the same frequency simultaneously, without interfering with each other's calls.

In order for you to operate a car phone, the trunk of your car will be equipped with a powerful minicomputer containing a built-in transmitter-receiver that recognizes your personal car code number. For an incoming call, all the grid-cell computers in your city would broadcast your code. Your computer would respond by notifying the closest grid computer of your location and then making the connection. All this takes place in a split second. If, for example, you are talking as you drive out of cell number 11 and into cell number 12, grid computer 11 would automatically relay the broadcasting responsibility to grid computer 12. This computer "handshake" occurs so quickly, your call is uninterrupted.

Although the system may sound complex, it is really elegantly simple, consisting of scores to hundreds of tiny grid computers "talking to" thousands of even smaller car computers. Once installed, a city's grid network would operate at lightning speed and without human operators. Motorola's Communications Group has already devised a plan that divides the Washington-Baltimore area into five hexagonal cells, each with an eleven-mile radius, and a similar system is being tested by American Telephone and Telegraph in Chicago. If tests during the early 1980s run smoothly, thousands of cars could be equipped with phones

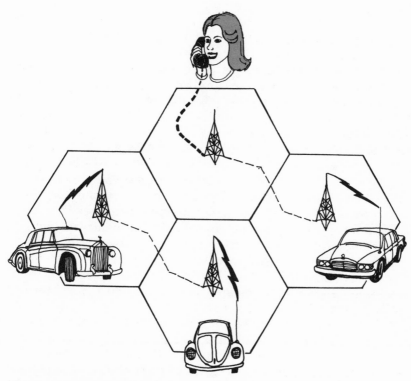

Communication Honeycomb

Sectioning cities into cells will make it possible for everyone to have a car phone. Computers will instantaneously relay calls as phones in operation leave one cell and enter an adjacent one.

by the end of the decade. Eventually, says AT&T's Thomas Nurnberger, the grid cell system will make it possible for virtually anyone on the move to have a telephone.

Home Computers

You may decide to plug your future phone into a small home computer. If you do, it could make life from the mid 1980s on a lot easier — and more fun.

You wake up late, it's raining heavily, and you have no time to do your important errands and still be ready for your dinner guests. So you rush to the phone and dial a special number that activates your computer's video screen or your television screen. The screen comes alive with an ad announcing department store sales, airline schedules, and the day's newspaper of your choice. At the computer keyboard you order and pay for that evening's meal, buy a dress, book the family's vacation flight to Florida, and electronically flip page by page through the newspaper without soiling your fingers. Sounds too good to be true? Well, a modified version of such a system, called Prestel, has been tested in thousands of homes in Britain, and by 1983 an estimated 5000 Americans in selected areas of the United States will be testing a similar service — the first home data-bank system in this country.

The heart of the system is the versatile home computer, which currently sells for about $3000. A marvel in its own right, a home computer can be programmed to balance your bank account, prepare your income tax return, or play video games; you can consult its "electronic encyclopedia" on how to prepare a low-cholesterol meal or repair a carburetor; or, by connecting your computer to your thermostat, you can save energy by turning down the hot-water heater between certain hours, turning off outside lights at sunrise, or keeping the air conditioner off until a half-hour before you arrive home. These various features are possible because of the home computer's formidable memory. But British scientists have advanced the concept of a home computer a significant step further, by linking home computers, via telephone lines, to a central computer agency. People thus can benefit from a variety of information and services that cannot fit into their home computer's memory.

Prestel's central computer agency holds more than 250,000 "electronic pages" of ads and services submitted periodically by stores, theaters, airlines, and travel agencies. In fact, shops specializing in everything from washing machines to wedding rings have submitted electronic pages to the central computer agency. A subscriber of Prestel scans the pages of interest to him (at a cost of three cents a page) and types his purchases on a keyboard, paying for them by punching his credit card number. Through Prestel, even electronic philanthropy is possible. The Save the Children charity has submitted a page urging Prestel subscribers to punch in the amount of their contributions. All purchases and contributions appear itemized on the subscribers' monthly telephone bills.

For all its versatility, the technology behind Prestel is very simple and has been used by department stores, the stock market, and theater-ticket agencies for years. Prestel, however, is the first system to bring this technology — and the features it offers — into the home. During the early 1980s, Prestel will be installed in additional British households at a very inexpensive monthly rate, since revenue from advertisers is expected to cover most of the service's overhead. The British have licensed U.S. rights for Prestel to the Insac Group, Inc., of New York, which expects to begin marketing the system in this country in the early 1980s. If gadget-hungry Americans adopt the system as enthusiastically as manufacturers anticipate, many of us could be doing our 1985 Christmas shopping from computer consoles in our homes.

· · ·

Even before home computers are linked with central computer agencies, technologists are planning the next step in computer living. By the 1990s they hope to have augmented the services made available to households through home computers by linking home computers, via telephone lines, directly with banks, department stores, and libraries. To take full advantage of the services these new hookups will permit, you will have to purchase a teleprinter device for your home that prints out information received over your telephone line. With a telephone–home computer–teleprinter system, here are some of the ways your life will be made easier in just another ten years.

Paying Bills

Linked to banks, home computers could render check-writing obsolete. With the system, you will be able to punch out the amount of each of the bills to be paid and watch your checking-account balance automatically decrease. For a slight fee your bank will make the payments you indicate.

Sending Letters

You could also send letters via your computer if the respondent has a computer. All you need do is dial the computer code number of the person to whom you're sending the message. As you type the letter at your keyboard it would appear instantaneously on the recipient's paper recorder. To prevent companies and charities that learn of your home computer code number from burdening you with reams of junk mail, flooding your living room with print-out, there may have to be strict laws against transmitting unsolicited mail over telephone lines.

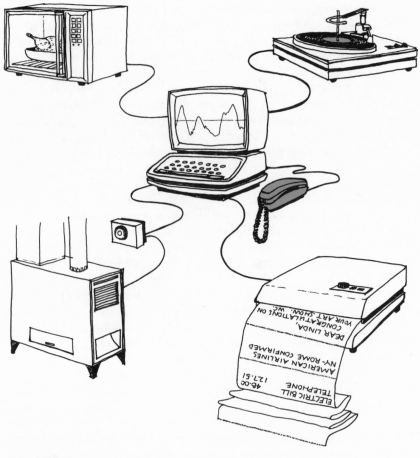

Easy Living

Every electrical and mechanical appliance in a home can be operated through a home computer. Here a teleprinter obviates the need for mail, since bills, reservations, and letters are transmitted over telephone lines and are printed in the recipient's home.

Library Borrowing

Connected to libraries, home computer video screens could display any book, journal, or newspaper that your library (or any library in the world) has stored on microfilm. A librarian, for instance, could insert the microfilm for a back edition of the *New York Times*, and with your computer controls you could advance the film as you would if you were actually in the library. To copy a particular article, you would simply press a control button and the library's microfilm system would photograph the article, transmit the information over telephone lines, and your teleprinter would reproduce the article. Pictures, too, could be sent and received by a similar process.

Purchasing Tickets

You would be able to consult your video screen for available seats in a theater or on a plane, or for hotel rooms, and then make a selection and type in your credit card number as payment. If your credit was good, your teleprinter would then print the equivalent of tickets or reservations, and it would be honored by the theater, airline, or hotel.

Dial a Doctor

Instead of visiting the doctor for a regular checkup, you may prefer to attach a medical device to your home computer that could serve the same purpose. The device would measure heart rate, blood pressure, and body temperature, and conduct complete urine and blood analyses — given samples of each — then submit the information via telephone line to your doctor or hospital for diagnosis.

You may even receive inexpensive psychotherapy for depression, phobias, or neuroses by tying into a "psychological" computer at a medical center. (See *Computer Diagnosis*, p. 215; and *Computer Therapy*, p. 217.) Computer experts project that by the end of this century home computers linked to public services will be considered not a luxury, but an absolute necessity for living in the twenty-first century.

Two-Way Television

By 1985 your television set could be connected to a revolutionary pay-cable system called Qube that allows subscribers a rich variety of programs — and the ability to talk back to politicians and television executives through what is being termed "interactive" television.

Although Qube offers a unique range of educational seminars, religious services, opera, and even soft-core pornography, what makes the system truly revolutionary is that it represents a first in two-way television. Information flows into and out of subscribers' homes over two-way cables that connect television sets to a central computer center. With a hand-held console the size of a large paperback, a subscriber can select channels, push "yes" and "no" buttons in response to questions flashed on the screen, and numerically rate shows. Qube is being test-marketed in Columbus, Ohio, where 20,000 households have subscribed to the system. Thus far, Columbus subscribers have voted on local and national political issues, their choice for the Academy Awards, and have registered complaints about the high cost of food. Subscribers have also used the cable system to purchase merchandise from television ads, to reserve tables in restaurants, and even to order their meals in advance.

If you become a Qube subscriber, however, you must be willing to relinquish a modicum of privacy, for, while you're watching Qube television, it's literally watching you. The central computer sweeps each subscribing household every six seconds, monitoring the programs being viewed. This capability of Qube has raised serious questions concerning invasion of privacy. Is it the business of the executives at Qube's central control to know whether you are watching an opera or a pornographic movie? Could a company attempting to gauge a prospective employee's cultural tastes or political opinions persuade or pressure central computer executives to release information about that person's viewing choices and voting records? In addition, Qube's potential to take instant political polls has many congressmen worried. "People will be giving their opinions even before they are informed on the issues," says Charles D. Ferris, chairman of the Federal Communications Commission. "No senator or congressman is going to go against what becomes publicly known about the consensus of his or her constituency."

The Qube marketing experiment in Columbus, however, has been so successful that Warner Communications, the marketer of Qube, plans to offer interactive television to residents of Akron and Pittsburgh in the early 1980s. There seems to be little doubt that two-way television will expand nationally. Media experts predict that two-way television will be in eight million homes by the late 1980s, and in fifty million homes by the end of this century. Before that can happen, however, the government must adopt regulations that balance First Amendment freedoms and invasion of privacy issues.

Neutrino Talk

The first message to be sent *through* the earth will be carried by ghostlike subatomic particles that are virtually without mass or electric charge. Neutrino broadcasts could revolutionize communications as profoundly as did Guglielmo Marconi's experiments in wireless telegraphy in the 1890s.

The neutrino is an ideal carrier of information. Its existence was postulated by Wolfgang Pauli in 1931, but it was discovered only in 1956. Twenty-five years passed between theory and discovery, because the physical properties of neutrinos are so nonexistent that the average neutrino can pass through all the matter in the universe without colliding with anything or slowing down or losing any appreciable energy. However, in a sufficiently intense beam of neutrinos, a tiny portion of the particles do collide with atoms in, say, a large body of water, producing tiny flashes.

At a cost of $120 million, the Naval Research Laboratory is developing a system called DUMAND (Deep Underwater Muon and Neutrino Detection), which depends on neutrino beams to communicate with deeply submerged missile submarines. This is a national-security problem that has defied conventional radio systems, since water effectively blocks out electromagnetic signals.

Muons, or, more technically, mu mesons, are more massive subatomic particles, each one 207 times the size of an electron and carrying an electric charge. Muons have nowhere near the penetrating power of neutrinos, but they can pass through thick steel plates and blocks of concrete. The first muon message was sent at the Argonne National Laboratory in April 1972; it passed through 1.5 yards of concrete and steel and was received 160 yards away. If the intensity of muon signals is increased, a beam could reach a maximum range of 500 miles.

A group of physicists headed by Dr. Peter Kotzer of Western Washington University hopes to send the first neutrino message from the 400-billion-electron-volt particle accelerator at the Fermi National Accelerator Laboratory in Batavia, Illinois. The beam will be directed downward at an angle of about 21 degrees, to pass through the earth and emerge in Puget Sound, 1707 miles away. The message will be encoded in a manner analogous to Morse code, and the entire one million tons of water in Puget Sound will serve as the detector-target. Showers of particles will be recorded each time a neutrino collides with a larger particle. The tiny flashes of light will subsequently be translated back into the original message. If Dr. Kotzer's plans proceed without a hitch, the first neutrino message could be sent by 1982.

Because of their penetrating power, neutrino beams could carry messages through deep space. "Applications of neutrino communications are enormous," says Dr. Kotzer. "Unless our conception of the nature of neutrinos at this point is seriously at fault, the system not only would work, it could revolutionize communications."

Hydrogen Talk

There could soon be a far more efficient way to transmit sound, visual images, and data than through conventional metal wires, which waste energy because of their resistance to electrical signals. The better communicator would be a kind of metal wire made from solidifying hydrogen gas under extreme pressure. Although the process for manufacturing hydrogen wire is still in the early stages of research, once perfected, wires and power lines made of metallic hydrogen could conduct electricity cross-country with no loss in energy, thereby saving millions of dollars annually. Hydrogen wires could also revolutionize the computer and electronics fields in the 1990s.

The modern alchemist's dream of transforming common hydrogen gas into a miracle metal is at least a hundred years old. As the lightest and simplest element in the universe, hydrogen is a member of the class of elements known as alkali metals, all of which (lithium, sodium, potassium, rubidium, cesium), except hydrogen, exist in a metallic state at room temperature. Physicists believe that hydrogen, too, under sufficiently extreme pressure could be forced to resemble its sister elements. And solid hydrogen would prove a superconducting metal, for in the process of producing it, the frenetic motion of its molecules — which offers resistance to electric signals — would be stilled (the hydrogen molecules actually split into individual atoms), thus allowing currents to pass unimpeded.

The belief that hydrogen gas could be transformed into a metal was given a major boost in 1979, when scientists at Cornell University demonstrated that under immense pressures the gas xenon coalesced into a superconducting metal. Xenon, however, is a rare element and could never be produced in large enough quantities for practical applications. Hydrogen, however, being one of the most abundant elements on earth, could have numerous applications as a superconducting metal.

Hard as Rubies

Two research teams, employing different methods, believe they may have produced small amounts of metallic hydrogen in pressurized chambers. Scientists at the United States Army's Watervliet Arsenal in New York chilled gaseous hydrogen into a liquid, then subjected the liquid to pressure 100,000 times greater than atmospheric pressure at sea level (100 kilobars). The scientists are testing their rock-hard hydrogen with sound waves and electrical currents for clues that would indicate the hydrogen has acquired the properties of a superconducting metal.

Scientists at the Geophysical Laboratory of the Carnegie Institute in Washington have had even greater success in solidifying hydrogen — and without the need for constant cooling. In 1979 they subjected hydrogen in a sealed chamber to an incredible pressure of 360 kilobars and produced, at room temperature (in the pressure chamber), a chunk of solid yellowish hydrogen that was as crystalline as sugar, as dense as rubies. Although their hydrogen is solid, it may not qualify as a superconducting metal, because modern physical theory posits that hydrogen gas won't become a permanent superconducting metal at room temperature unless a pressure of 1000 kilobars is achieved.

The Carnegie and army teams both hope that once hydrogen metal is formed and removed from its pressure chamber, it will not instantly evaporate into its gaseous state. This is an essential requirement, of course, for metallic hydrogen to be used as a practical substance. Scientists remain optimistic that they will attain the required 1000 kilobars of pressure in a few years and that by the end of this century companies will be extracting hydrogen from the world's oceans to produce extraordinarily efficient power lines.

21

Energy Breakthroughs:
Power from the Sun
–and Just About Everything Under It

Wind, sea, crop wastes, percolating plasmas, and giant satellites that beam the sun's energy to earth in the form of microwaves represent but a few of the energy sources that will supplant the world's dwindling supplies of oil and natural gas over the next several decades. The United States Department of Energy is spending over $300 million a year investigating these alternate energy sources, in an attempt to break the country's dependence on foreign oil.

It is clear that no single source of energy can meet the world's future energy needs. A combination of power sources, however, would go a long way toward extending the life of our precious natural resources, a fact that is increasingly important, given the current uncertain status of nuclear power. Many of the energy schemes for the 1980s and beyond are elegantly simple; others are so exotic, they stretch the boundaries of technology. All of them, though, are designed to be as pollution-free as possible.

Gasoal

Coal is to the United States what oil is to the Middle East. Beneath the continental United States lie at least a trillion tons of coal, enough to last several hundred years, if consumed at the present rate. Hard coal, unfortunately, is not an ideal energy source; gas and oil, though scarcer, are far cleaner and more convenient to use. Coal, however, is produced from the same prehistoric plant and animal remains as gas and oil, so theoretically it should be possible to convert coal into gas and oil.

Coal differs from gas and oil in one respect: coal has less of the combustible element hydrogen. For coal to be converted to gas or oil, then, its hydrogen content must be increased. This is precisely what companies such as Mobil and Exxon are doing to produce the equivalent of natural gas, and gasoal, a liquid with the color, smell, and combustible behavior of gasoline that could be powering our cars by the 1990s.

Each oil company has developed its own conversion process, but the schemes are basically similar. First, the coal is pulverized and transformed under heat into either a crude gas or liquid; then it is mixed with hydrogen under pressure. The product is either commercial gas or oil, depending on the amount of hydrogen added to the coal and the length of time the mixture is allowed to simmer. At an experimental plant Exxon is currently producing 3 barrels of oil a day from 1 ton of coal, and the company has a 250-ton-a-day plant under construction outside Houston, Texas. Ashland Oil Company has completed a pilot plant in Kentucky capable of converting 600 tons of coal daily into 2200 barrels of crude oil that can then be refined to yield commercial gas.

The technology for converting coal to oil and gas is not new. In an experimental project in the 1940s government scientists converted 500 pounds of coal into 13 gallons of gasoal at a cost of about nineteen cents a gallon. At that time gasoline sold for seventeen cents a gallon, so the gasoal experiment was abandoned. Currently, it costs ninety cents to produce a gallon of gasoal, and that figure is expected to be reduced to seventy-five cents by the mid-to-late 1980s — thereby making gasoal competitive with, if not cheaper than, gasoline. Since gasoal has a lower octane rating than standard petroleum-derived gasoline, researchers predict that cars in the next decade may run on fifty-fifty blends of gasoal and gasoline — a clean, inexpensive fuel that will stretch our petroleum reserves.

Before that goal can be realized, however, scientists must solve the problem of producing large quantities of gasoal without polluting the environment in the process of preparing coal for the conversion process. Fortunately, coal-cleaning technology is progressing so rapidly that the large oil companies are betting that before the end of the century cars will be powered with gasoal blends and that gasoal in its liquid form will be used to heat homes inexpensively.

Biofuels

Agricultural wastes and urban garbage make up a vast potential source of energy that may one day provide our energy-starved world with an inexhaustible supply of fuel. The world produces 100 million tons of biomass — biological and biodegradable material — a year, enough to satisfy the energy requirements of the United States six times over. Scientists are busy devising methods for extracting this latent energy in the form of alcohol and methane gas.

The principle behind converting biomass to biofuel is relatively simple. Trapped inside every plant is solar energy in the form of sugars, mostly glucose, that have been manufactured during the process of photosynthesis. Just as glucose powers our bodies, it can also be transformed, when fermented with yeasts, into two types of alcohol to power cars: methanol (or wood alcohol, which is poisonous to the body), and ethanol (the essence of spirits). The potential of alcohol as a fuel has been known for years. In fact, alcohol powered many of Henry Ford's early cars, and to this day Indianapolis racing cars run on almost pure alcohol. In recent tests in Germany, scientists ran forty-five vehicles nearly a million miles on fuel composed of 15 percent alcohol and 85 percent gasoline — a mixture referred to as gasohol — and the cars performed perfectly in all kinds of weather conditions.

To date, widespread use of gasohol has been impeded by the cost and technological difficulty of extracting glucose from plant cellulose. But recent breakthroughs are about to make the production of gasohol easier and less costly. Dr. George Tsao of Purdue University is perfecting an extraction process that could yield commercial, clean-burning alcohol for about eighty cents a gallon. The Tsao process begins by dissolving wheat, corn, potatoes, sugar beets — any plant with a high starch or sugar content — in a dilute sulfuric-acid bath to remove the outer cell wall. Two plant fibers that are chemically bound — lignin and cellulose — remain. This mixture is then neutralized with lime, dried, and sloshed violently about in a tumbler of more highly concentrated sulfuric acid to dissolve the bonds between the lignin and cellulose, thus producing pulp cellulose. The pulp is washed, dried, then bathed with a final acid bath to extract the valuable glucose. The solid lignin by-product can be burned to provide heat and power for the biofuel refinery, and the glucose is funneled into huge vats, where it's fermented into pure, high-energy ethanol, or methanol by use of a slightly different process. In laboratory experiments, Tsao has been able to convert 90 percent of a plant's cellulose into glucose in just one hour. With the help of a $2 million dollar grant from the state of Indiana, Tsao expects to perfect his process by 1982 and to have compiled enough data to enable a commercial firm to construct an actual biomass refinery.

Gasohol in Operation

Despite the present cost of alcohol, some areas of the United States are already selling gasohol. In 1978, 100,000 gallons of gasohol were sold in Nebraska, and in 1979 consumers in the Plains states bought 900,000 gallons of gasohol. The Environmental Protection Agency has already given permission for service stations to sell gasohol as a substitute for unleaded gas. Senator Birch Bayh, chairman of the recently formed National Alcohol Fuels Commission, says, "We need capital investment to exploit distillation processes already developed that would produce twice as much alcohol for half the price. With the use of ten million acres of farmland now out of production, we then would see plant scientists coming up with crops of BTUs [energy] rather than proteins."

As it happens, Brazil is doing just that — cultivating crops specifically for their energy content. Brazil is well on its way to becoming the first country to replace conventional fuels with gasohol and alcohol. By taking advantage of their country's vast sugar cane crop, Brazilians are powering most of their cars and buses with gasohol mixtures. By 1985, Brazil plans to extract enough alcohol from sugar cane to replace a fifth of the country's annual gasoline consumption. And by the 1990s, Brazilian officials hope most of the country's vehicles will be operating on pure alcohol alone.

Alcohol, however, is not the only biofuel that can be extracted from biomass. The Calorific Recovery Anaerobic Process, Inc., in Oklahoma is converting animal wastes into methane gas. The process involves stripping vast quantities of cattle waste of its fibrous content and mixing it in tanks with bacteria that thrive on waste. The bacterial decomposition process releases ammonia, carbon dioxide, and methane gas — as much as 1.6 million cubic feet a day from the waste of 100,000 cattle. The plant expects to start selling its methane gas to consumers by the early 1980s.

The unique advantage of biofuels — or, as they're also called, home-grown fuels — is that their source, plants, is inexhaustible. Researchers predict a time when biomass refineries will have spread across the country to receive every day farms' corn stalks and harvest stubble, cities' wastes, and lumber companies' wood scraps and to convert these materials into biofuels for powering cars and heating homes. Slightly further in the future, "energy farms" may become a reality — farms where fast-growing crops like sugar cane, sorghum, and sugar beets will be raised solely for their usable energy.

Wind Power

By the end of this century the coastline of the United States and the country's interior windy plains could be dotted with brightly colored windmills capable of producing sizable amounts of electric power. But because the wind can be a gale or a zephyr, the federal government plans to design windmill systems that take into account the wind's capriciousness. The task is challenging, but the rewards incalculable. Wind power is cleaner than the air that produces it, completely safe, and very economical.

The first in a line of windmills the Department of Energy will construct during the 1980s was built recently in Clayton, New Mexico. Bearing little resemblance to traditional Dutch windmills, the Clayton whirler has two 63-foot orange, white, and blue blades that rotate to spin a turbine whenever wind speeds exceed eight miles an hour. The $1 million windmill has proved that it can feed enough electricity into the local power grid to supply 60 of the town's 1300 homes with energy. Since its construction, similar 200-kilowatt windmills have begun operating on Block Island, Rhode Island; and Culebra Island, Puerto Rico. A 2000-kilowatt generator with 100-foot blades is also working near Boone, North Carolina. The largest windmill project in the United States will be constructed in the early 1980s by U.S. Windpower, Inc., of Massachusetts. The company plans to build twenty 150-foot-high windmills in California's gusty Pacheco Pass, eighty miles south of San Francisco. When completed, the windmills are expected to supply enough power for 1000 people and save 175,000 barrels of oil a year.

In a variation on the DOE's model, Danish scientists have built the world's most powerful windmill, consisting of three 89-feet-long fiber-glass blades atop a 175-foot tower that produces four million kilowatt-hours of electricity a year. (A windmill's generating capacity is not determined by the number of its blades, but by the diameter of the rotor to which the blades are attached.) Danish scientists estimate that 1100 such windmills could supply enough electricity to satisfy 20 percent of Denmark's current energy needs.

Naturally, not every city or town has the ideal average wind speeds — between eight to thirty-five miles an hour — necessary to generate windmill electricity. In the United States, a ten-year National Weather Service study to determine regional speeds uncovered several surprises. Chicago, long called the Windy City, actually ranks tenth among cities having wind speeds that would make windmills practical. (The highest winds in the United States are at Mount Washington in New Hampshire, where the average speed is an attractive 34 miles an hour — but where maximum winds often exceeding 100 miles an hour could easily rip the blades off a windmill). Some cities ripe for the windmills in the 1980s are:

	Average Wind Speed
Fargo, North Dakota	14.4 mph
Wichita, Kansas	13.7
Boston, Massachusetts	13.3
New York, New York	12.9
Fort Worth, Texas	12.5
Des Moines, Iowa	12.1
Honolulu, Hawaii	12.1
Milwaukee, Wisconsin	12.1
Cleveland, Ohio	11.6
Chicago, Illinois	11.2
Minneapolis, Minnesota	11.2
Indianapolis, Indiana	10.8
Providence, Rhode Island	10.7
Seattle-Tacoma, Washington	10.7
San Francisco, California	10.6
Baltimore, Maryland	10.4
Detroit, Michigan	10.3
Denver, Colorado	10.0
Kansas City, Missouri	9.8
Atlanta, Georgia	9.7
Washington, D.C.	9.7
Philadelphia, Pennsylvania	9.6
Portland, Maine	9.6
New Orleans, Louisiana	9.0
Miami, Florida	8.8
Little Rock, Arkansas	8.7
Salt Lake City, Utah	8.7
Albuquerque, New Mexico	8.6
Tucson, Arizona	8.1
Birmingham, Alabama	7.9

Theoretically, it is possible to recover only about 60 percent of the kinetic energy, or energy of motion, in the wind. (To extract 100 percent of the wind's energy would require bringing all the wind in the vicinity of a windmill to a dead stop.) Yet even this 60 percent should be sufficient to supplement the energy needs of large sections of the United States. The Department of Energy estimates that if wind power is responsible for just 1 percent of the nation's energy, it could reduce imported-oil bills by millions of dollars.

Currently, it costs about three times as much to generate electricity from windmills as from oil, but the cost is expected to be more reasonable as the size of windmills increases. The capriciousness of the wind does not have to be a problem, since most windmills are being designed to link up with existing power resources on calm, windless days. Many energy experts forecast that by the year 2000 large areas of the United States will be picturesquely dotted with attractive, noiseless, pollution-free windmills spinning out as much as 10 percent of the country's electrical-energy needs.

Sea Power

Harnessing the energy of ocean waves has been a dream of visionary thinkers for more than 300 years. But only recently has technology been able to bring that dream within the realm of reality. During the late 1980s two sea-energy breakthroughs are expected: tidal power, a technique that generates power by using the tremendous mechanical energy in waves and the ebb and flow of tides; and ocean thermal-energy conversion, a process that generates energy from the temperature differences between the ocean's relatively warm surface and its chilly depths.

Tidal Power

To extract the mechanical energy in waves, scientists envision employing rows of giant buoys that bob up and down with the waves. Each would be connected to a crank; the cranks would rotate the blades of a generator that could drive a turbine to produce electricity. Studies are underway to locate the best gulfs, inlets, and coastal stretches for tapping the sea's energy. Cook Inlet in Alaska and Passamaquoddy Bay in Maine are slated for experimental tidal power plants in the early 1980s. According to one federal study, commercial-size plants at these two sites could churn almost twenty billion kilowatt-hours of electricity, enough to meet the needs of a state the size of Colorado.

American scientists are also studying British and Japanese tidal power plant designs. In August 1978 a floating, 500-ton experimental station located 2.5 miles off Japan's Honshu Island began producing 125 kilowatts of power. The facility is unique in that it contains several cylindrical air chambers jutting into the sea and housing large floats. The floats bob with passing waves, forcing air through vents in the tops of the chambers, and this pressurized air, in turn, propels turbines that generate electric power. British scientists have taken another approach to capturing wave power with their ingenious concept of "contour rafts," which resemble huge butterflies. Three rectangular rafts are hinged together by cylinders containing pistons. Waves rock the rafts, flexing the hinges and forcing the pistons to pump water, and this water propels turbines that produce electricity. Small versions of the contour rafts floating in the English Channel have demonstrated that the system is highly efficient, and its designer, Sir Christopher Cockerell, inventor of the Hovercraft, claims that 300 of the mechanical butterflies batting their wings could generate as much energy as a conventional power station. In a few years scientists expect to have collected sufficient data on the operation of the American buoy, the Japanese float, and the British butterfly — as well as on other techniques — to determine the best tidal power plant design.

Ocean Thermal-Energy Conversion

An alternative approach to harnessing sea power treats the ocean as a giant battery that is recharged (heated) daily by the sun. To produce power, the process takes advantage of the 30°-to-40° temperature difference of water at the ocean surface and at depths of about 2000 to 3000 feet. Warm water from the ocean surface is used to heat a low-boiling-point liquid coolant like ammonia into pressurized vapor; the vapor, in turn, drives an electrical generator the same way as steam drives turbines in a conventional steam generator. In the second step of the operation, colder water from the ocean depths is raised through pipes to cool the vapor back to its original liquid form. The entire process is then repeated. Thus, the ocean's temperature differential — caused by the sun — is harnessed to do the work of driving turbines. In effect, the OTEC process is extracting the solar energy stored in vast quantities in the world's oceans.

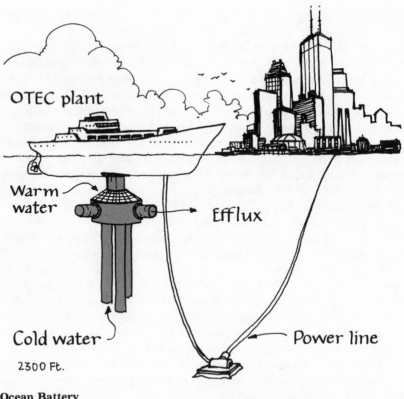

OTEC plant

Warm water

Efflux

Cold water

Power line

2300 Ft.

Ocean Battery

Temperature differences between sun-warmed surface water and colder water at a depth of more than 2000 feet are used to generate electricity for coastal cities.

Initial attempts to extract large amounts of energy with the OTEC process have begun off the coast of Hawaii, eighteen miles northwest of Ke-Ahole Point. There, the sun-heated water-surface temperatures range from 75° to 82° Fahrenheit, compared with a 41° Fahrenheit water temperature 2300 feet below the surface. For the experiment, a navy tanker has been converted into a floating OTEC power plant. Three pipes, each four feet in diameter, hang from beneath the ship to draw cold water from the ocean depths. This federal project, costing $43 million and dubbed OTEC-1, is expected to generate one million watts of electric power in the early 1980s. If OTEC-1 proves as successful as scientists anticipate, several major companies are ready to begin construction of their own experimental OTEC plants. Many energy experts predict that in fifteen years hundreds of floating OTEC plants, linked to shore by underwater transmission lines, could be anchored around the coast of the United States, each plant capable of producing 100 million watts of power.

Hot-Rock Power

Scientists once estimated that the use of geothermal energy was restricted to those few areas of the world fortunate enough to be located over primordial underground hot springs. In the United States, Utah, Nevada, and Idaho have geothermal power plants, and the Geysers, a geothermal site in northern California, has for a number of years been using subterranean steam to produce 400 megawatts of electricity for the power lines of the Pacific Gas and Electric Company — enough to supply more than half the energy required by the city of San Francisco.

Within the last few years, geologists have discovered potentially vast sources of a different kind of "low-temperature" geothermal energy. Fortunately, such sources exist in the populous eastern region of the United States, where energy is most needed. In addition, scientists are experimenting with two ways to create their own geothermal sites. They are pumping water into super-hot volcanic rocks, and, in areas that do not have natural underground volcanism, they are setting off nuclear explosions to ignite rocks before dousing them, saunalike, with water. Combining all these sources, proponents of geothermal power project a total output from geothermal plants of up to 20,000 megawatts by 1985 and perhaps as much as 400,000 megawatts by the end of this century — or 40 percent of the United States' total electric needs at that time. We shall witness the development of these new types of geothermal energy during the 1980s and 1990s.

Low-Temperature Geothermal Energy

In the western United States steam from geothermal wells is sufficiently hot to permit the economical production of electricity. However, the potential geothermal sites in eastern states such as New Jersey, Maryland, and Georgia probably contain geothermal heat that is too cool for inexpensive electrical production — but ideal for heating and air conditioning homes, offices, greenhouses, and for running hot-water systems. Geologists estimate that beneath the eastern states exist numerous spongelike sandstone formations containing water at a tepid 200° to 300° Fahrenheit. Engineers of the Department of Energy plan to drill into the sandstone and recover the hot water. The heat will be extracted from the water by mixing the water with a "working fluid" — a chemical similar to isobutane, which is immiscible with water and readily boils to produce the steam necessary to drive turbines.

Experimental wells sunk throughout the East Coast have shown areas along the southern New Jersey coast; Norfolk, Virginia; Wilmington, North Carolina; Charleston, South Carolina; and Savannah, Georgia, to be the prime candidates for future geothermal power plants. DOE engineers expect that by the late 1980s thousands of people on the East Coast will be heating and cooling their homes with geothermal power, cutting their energy bills and saving the country millions of dollars in oil imports.

Manmade Geothermal Wells

Somewhat further in the future lies the auspicious possibility of creating geothermal wells where none naturally exists. This could be accomplished by splitting underground rocks heated naturally by volcanic activity deep in the earth and then pumping in water to produce steam. Progress in this area is being reported by scientists at Los Alamos, New Mexico. They have fractured superhot granite two miles inside the earth with dynamite blasts, then drilled two holes about 250 feet apart and pumped water down one of these holes to circulate throughout the hot rocks. Through connecting fissures in the rock bed, the superheated water, tremendously pressurized, reaches the second, or venting, hole, where it percolates to the surface and flashes into steam capable of driving electric generators.

Research with manmade geothermal wells is still in its early stages. But scientists suspect that these artificial wells will yield more power than natural wells, because their rocks have not come into contact with underground water for centuries. These dry, hot rocks are as primed to release their energy to a splash of cold water as is a hot skillet on the stove. Such volcanically heated rock formations are thought to be abundant throughout the western United States, and by the end of this century could be used to double the amount of electricity generated by geothermal power plants.

Manmade geothermal wells may also be created in the central

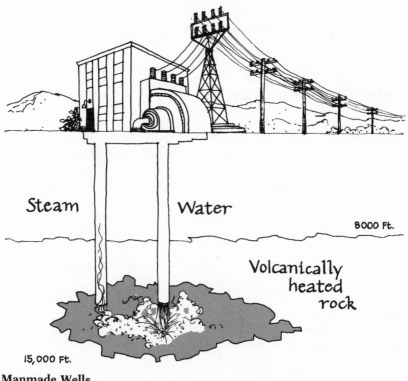

Steam   Water

8000 Ft.

Volcanically
heated
rock

15,000 Ft.

Manmade Wells

Dynamite blasts are used to create a cavity in hot granite rock. The rocks' heat (that is, energy) is captured — and extracted — when cold water is transformed into superhot steam.

and eastern parts of the country, if scientists involved with the controversial Project Pacer have their way. These nuclear scientists are exploring the possibility of detonating nuclear explosions deep in natural rock beds, thus creating superhot rocks and potential geothermal sites. Once the pumped-in water robbed the rocks of their peak heat, another nuclear blast would reheat them, recharging their generating capacity. The rocks, however, cool quickly. Judging by current calculations, for such an artificially created geothermal site to produce energy continuously, 10-kiloton nuclear blasts must be detonated every ten hours. Environmentalists rightly fear that radioactivity would be released in the escaping steam, but a more immediate danger could come from manmade earthquakes. Scientists will have at least two decades to examine these problems, for nuclear-heated geothermal wells are not expected to become a reality until the first quarter of the next century — if they materialize at all.

Solar Power Satellites

A satellite the size of Manhattan Island could be orbiting the earth by the turn of this century, collecting solar energy and beaming it to a field of receiving antennas in upstate New York. The resulting power would be sufficient to satisfy all of New York City's electric energy requirements. This futuristic concept, proposed in 1968 by Dr. Peter Glaser of Arthur D. Little, Inc., Cambridge, Massachusetts, is attracting the serious attention of scientists and the federal government. NASA and the Department of Energy are deep into a $16 million study that could result in the launching of an experimental solar power satellite (SPS) by 1990.

As presently conceived, solar power satellites would orbit 22,400 miles high and travel at the same speed as the earth, thus remaining fixed over one geographic location. Unencumbered by earth's atmosphere, an SPS's huge panel of solar cells — measuring as much as thirty miles wide by sixty miles long — would intercept sunlight in space with high efficiency for almost twenty-four hours a day. (A satellite in a geosynchronous orbit would be briefly eclipsed by the moon each day, reducing its solar power–collecting time by about fifteen minutes every twenty-four hours.) From earth the satellite would look to the naked eye at night like a bright star — a star that may also be faintly visible in daylight hours. The satellite's solar cells would convert sunlight directly to electricity. An onboard transducer would then convert the electricity to microwaves, which would be beamed to earth onto a field of receiving antennas covering an area the size of several football fields. Since microwaves are virtually unabsorbed as they pass through the earth's atmosphere, the energy beamed down by the satellite could be converted to electricity on earth with a high efficiency of 82 percent. A single SPS in geosynchronous orbit could produce 5 billion watts of electric power — a tremendous amount of energy, especially when we realize that a large power plant generates about 1.2 billion watts, and the peak power demands of New York City total 8 billion watts.

Many energy experts argue that the numerous advantages of SPSs more than justify the estimated $60 billion for research and development necessary to make the satellites a reality by the end

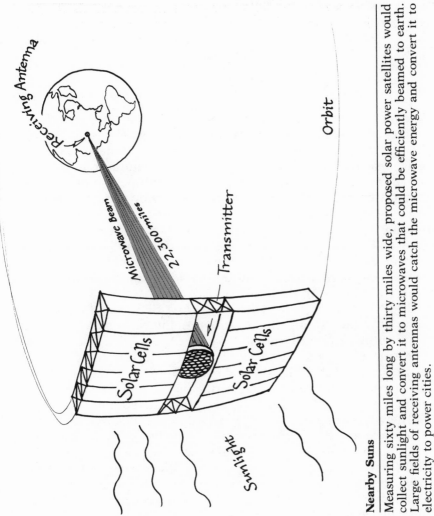

Nearby Suns

Measuring sixty miles long by thirty miles wide, proposed solar power satellites would collect sunlight and convert it to microwaves that could be efficiently beamed to earth. Large fields of receiving antennas would catch the microwave energy and convert it to electricity to power cities.

of this century. SPSs would tap a very nearly limitless source of energy and transmit that energy night and day, even during cloudy weather, eliminating the need for energy-storage facilities. Because of the high efficiency of converting solar energy into commercial electricity, the cost of such electricity would be relatively inexpensive — anywhere from two cents to fifteen cents a kilowatt-hour, compared with the current price of about twelve cents a kilowatt-hour. What's more, proponents argue that solar power satellites present no radiation threat.

Safety Factors

The microwave beams from SPSs would be aimed so precisely at the earth-based receiving antennas that even people living around the power plant would not be exposed to danger. Microwave leakage, experts claim, would remain within international standards of ten milliwatts per square centimeter imposed for microwave ovens. Even plane passengers flying through a microwave beam would be safe, protected by the plane's metal shielding and by the brief time spent in the rays. Peter Glaser has designed a fail-safe device so that if an SPS lost its lock on its earth-based antennas, the microwave beam would immediately spread out harmlessly in space. To protect birds, large screen fences would sheath the antenna fields.

The NASA–DOE plan envisions the first SPS being ferried into orbit by a space shuttle in the late 1980s. But the jumbo SPSs that could provide electric power for entire cities would have to be constructed in space. Under one plan to execute that construction, hundreds of workers would travel by space shuttle to a way station in a low orbit around earth; they would commute daily from the way station to the site of construction of the SPS.

There are, of course, many issues to be resolved before a scheme as ambitious and costly as a ring of solar power satellites becomes a reality. Mainly, will the microwave beams from many SPSs have an adverse heating effect on the earth's atmosphere? Will the beams interfere with a plane's navigation and communications? And, most important, can we be sure that stray microwave radiation will not affect plant, animal, and human life? We should have some of the answers by the end of the decade; then a serious commitment for construction of the satellites could begin. Many of the most respected aerospace scientists support the SPS program, and Dr. Glaser optimistically forecasts that by the year 2025, 100 solar power satellites will be suspended in orbit around the earth, providing at least 30 percent of the electrical energy needs of the United States.

Plasma Power

A sophisticated twenty-year-old technology known as magnetohydrodynamics (MHD) holds the promise of converting heat directly to electricity with very high efficiency. The process could provide the world with a new, inexpensive source of electric power for the 1990s.

The MHD process is based on a simple concept. A gas is superheated to several thousand degrees Fahrenheit. At this temperature, its neutrally charged molecules are converted into positive and negative ions, and the gas is transformed into a plasma. In an MHD generator, the hot plasma is blown through a magnetic field, where the energetic positive and negative ions are deflected to different electrodes and collected there, thus establishing an electric current. These basic principles have been familiar since the 1830s, when Michael Faraday described the behavior of electrically charged particles in a magnetic field. But the technology needed to contain a wildly energetic plasma in the gossamer boundaries of a magnetic field was not developed until the 1960s, and it's taken an additional twenty years for scientists to construct a prototype of a commercial MHD power plant. On December 6, 1977, near Moscow, a jointly owned United States–Soviet MHD experimental plant began producing electricity and sending it into the Moscow power grid. It was only a start, but that breakthrough convinced many scientists of the feasibility of electricity generated by the MHD process.

An MHD generator has many advantages over conventional power generators. The fact that an MHD generator has no moving parts means that it can operate at the ultrahigh temperatures necessary to make the conversion of heat to electricity efficient and economical — temperatures that would destroy the metals and lubricants in any conventional turbine. Current studies show that in converting heat to electric power, MHD generators are about 50 to 60 percent more efficient than fossil fuel plants, 30 percent more efficient than coal-fired generators, and about 25 percent more efficient than nuclear power plants. Conversion efficiency is important now and crucial for the future. According to a prediction by the Department of Energy, by the year 2000 half of the energy consumed in the United States may be used for the generation of electric power. If this calculation is correct, electric

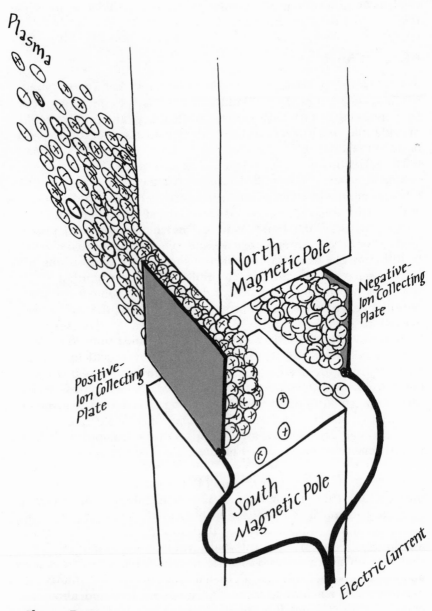

Plasma

North Magnetic Pole

Negative-Ion Collecting Plate

Positive-Ion Collecting Plate

South Magnetic Pole

Electric Current

Cleaner Power

A superhot ionized gas, or plasma, passed through a magnetic field produces clean electricity. Experimental plants are already producing respectable amounts of electric power, and commercial MDH plants may be only eight years away.

power plant designs must be more efficient than they now are. If they are not changed, the plants would waste one third of the energy consumed by the country — a waste equal to more than eight billion barrels of oil a year, at a cost of $120 billion!

It should be understood that this seemingly sinful waste is not due to the sloppy design and engineering of current power plants so much as to a fundamental principle of thermodynamics which states that the optimal efficiency of *any* heat engine is determined by the range of temperatures over which it operates. Thus, MHD is highly efficient because it operates at temperatures of several thousand degrees.

Unfortunately, these same high temperatures also mean that MHD plants will produce more noxious nitrous oxides. However, environmentalists agree that MHD's single major disadvantage is outweighed by many advantages. The exhaust from an MHD plant contains no soot, and because of their high overall efficiency, MHD generators release less waste heat into the environment. (The thermal pollution of lakes and rivers caused by the discharge of hot condenser-cooling water from conventional fossil fuel and nuclear plants is a major and growing environmental problem.)

It may be another decade before the technology for constructing MHD plants is perfected. But the continued success of the experimental United States–Soviet MHD plant has encouraged scientists. The Russians expect to complete a 500-megawatt MHD power plant in 1984, and the U.S. Department of Energy foresees construction of its own plant a few years later. MHD will not constitute a primary source of power by the end of this decade, but it will contribute measurably to efficient electricity generation in the future.

Harnessing Fusion

There is a major experiment in nuclear fusion scheduled to occur at Princeton University in the 1980s, and it is expected to herald the dawn of the golden age of almost limitless amounts of energy for the twenty-first century. By taming nuclear fusion, physicists will have realized a fifty-year-old dream and have achieved the biggest single energy breakthrough in history.

Fusion is the energy process that fires the sun, and it's one of nature's cleverest tricks. When two hydrogen nuclei unite, they form a particle whose mass is less than the sum of the original particles. This tiny mass difference is released as a tremendous burst of energy, as was shown by Einstein's celebrated formula $E = mc^2$. As a source of energy, fusion has dramatic advantages over the controversial fission process employed by nuclear power plants. Fusion produces almost no radioactive wastes, whereas fission generates troublesome piles of plutonium, which must be safely disposed of underground, at sea, or in space. More important, fusion is fueled by hydrogen, the most abundant element in the sea.

However, harnessing the energy produced when two hydrogen nuclei fuse together has proved a monumental technical task. To attain fusion, a plasma of volatile hydrogen nuclei must be confined securely, squeezed to enormous density, and heated to a critical temperature of 100 million degrees Celsius. A vital step toward achieving that goal occurred at the Princeton Plasma Physics Laboratory in August 1978. For a fleeting twenty milliseconds, the doughnut-shaped contraption known as the Princeton Large Torus held a plasma of hydrogen nuclei and its isotope, deuterium, in a strong magnetic field, or "magnetic bottle," at a temperature of 60 million degrees Celsius — four times higher than the sun's own internal heat. (A temperature of 100 million degrees Celsius is required to initiate a fusion reaction, but once begun, the fusion process can continue at lower temperatures.)

Despite the brevity of the Princeton reaction, it lasted long enough to assure physicsts of the scientific feasibility of fusion power. The success at Princeton has encouraged physicists at the Sandia Laboratory in Albuquerque, New Mexico, and the Lawrence Livermore Laboratory in California who are working on equally promising approaches to nuclear fusion: the use of "magnetic mirrors" to concentrate hydrogen plasma in a long cylinder, and the employment of laser beams to bombard tiny hydrogen fuel pellets to create high-density matter at ultrahigh temperatures.

Of course, the real success of harnessing fusion power will depend on physicists being able to attain a temperature of 100 million degrees Celsius and reaching that magical break-even point at which the energy output of a fusion reaction equals the energy input. Princeton scientists expect to have a new, bigger torus in operation by 1981. Melvin Gottlieb, who heads the Plasma Physics Laboratory, believes that this tighter magnetic bottle will contain the fusion reaction securely enough to attain the break-even point some time in the mid-to-late 1980s. So we're about thirty years away from enjoying the benefits of commercial fusion power plants. But that wait will be handsomely rewarded. Researchers in the field of fusion power agree that, in theory, no single energy source has more potential than nuclear fusion for powering the world in the twenty-first century and beyond.

Glassy Solar Cells

Currently, an estimated 100,000 American families rely on solar energy to heat their water, and even fewer use solar energy to heat their homes. In the next two decades, however, the utilization of solar energy should jump dramatically, due to the development of inexpensive solar cells that devour sunlight on one side and produce electricity on the other. It appears that this breakthrough will come from a new class of versatile compounds known as glassy solar cells, or amorphous semiconductors. And according to the optimistic estimates, this breakthrough may occur by the mid-to-late 1980s, transforming the solar cell from an exotic, expensive space-age device to into an inexpensive, everyday workhorse.

The first solar cell was developed by Bell Laboratory scientists several decades ago in the form of a silicon crystal; it employed the principles of solid state physics to convert sunlight directly into electricity. Since that time, silicon crystal solar cells have been used extensively as power sources in satellites and spacecraft. But the high cost of manufacturing these precision crystals has never dropped low enough to encourage their commercial use. Silicon solar cells currently cost about $10 per peak watt (the cell's energy output at high noon on a cloudless day), and a panel of physicists reported to the Department of Energy in 1979 that the cost of silicon solar cells is unlikely to drop below fifty cents per peak watt at any time in the future. To compete with coal-fired and nuclear power plants, solar cells would have to cost about ten to twenty cents per peak watt. Remarkably, the new glassy solar cells may be able to convert sunlight to electricity for about half the cost.

Present-day solar cells consist of rows of perfectly aligned atoms of silicon laced with so-called doping elements, which permit electric current to flow. As their name implies, amorphous semiconductors are jumbles of atoms with no particular pattern, like ordinary window glass. Because of their random molecular structure, such materials were considered almost useless until an independent inventor, Stanford Ovshinsky, startled the world of solid state physics in the 1960s with the claim that he had constructed a functioning solar cell basically of inexpensive, amorphous glass. After their initial skepticism, several scientists began experimenting with glassy materials and soon demonstrated that it was precisely the materials' jumbled molecular structures that produced unexpected, complex chemical bonds that aid in the conduction of electricity. Scientists are still not exactly sure how amorphous materials work, but amorphous-glass research received a valuable boost in 1977 when the Nobel physics prize was awarded to three physicists for their fundamental studies relating to glassy semiconductors.

Present-day silicon solar cells must be meticulously manufactured and then mounted with great care on the exterior of a spacecraft or house roof — often at great expense. Amorphous solar cells, however, could be constructed and mounted on a house roof as a do-it-yourself weekend project. For example, thin sheets of ordinary steel would be mounted on the southern façade of a house. They would then be sprayed with a special fast-drying liquid that formed a thin glassy film in which two wires would be embedded before the film hardened. The wires would conduct the direct current produced by the film-steel sandwich to a standard device that would convert direct current into alternating current for use in the home's electrical system.

Ovshinsky's marvelous spray does not yet exist, but it could by the end of the deacde. Scientists are convinced that glassy solar cells will play a role in powering tomorrow's homes. Following Ovshinsky's lead, Exxon and Mobil are creating their own glassy solar cell designs, and RCA scientists are perfecting an amorphous material that, when squeezed between two plates of ordinary glass, converts sunlight to electricity. The RCA solar cell may be commercially available by the 1990s.

Ovshinsky predicts that once the technology is developed, the cost of amorphous solar cells could sink to as low as five cents per peak watt, making solar-generated electricity the cheapest kind. Theoretically, we know that the sunlight falling on the earth could provide 100,000 times the total energy output of all existing power plants. By the 1990s, store-bought solar cells and do-it-yourself spray cells could begin capturing part of that energy.

Superbulbs

Imagine a 100-watt light bulb that consumes only 40 watts of electricity. It may sound impossible, but such bulbs may be lighting homes by the mid 1980s. These superbulbs could reduce a home's energy consumption by 60 percent while producing the full

Coating transmits visible light and reflects heat back to filament.

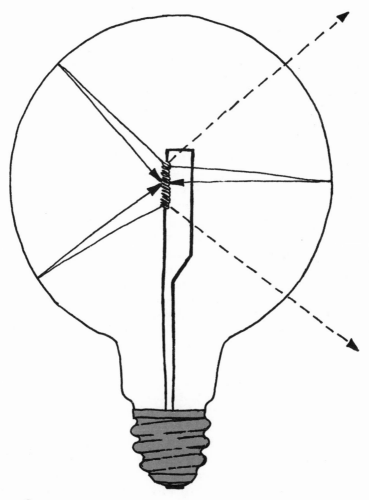

Energy Saver

By utilizing heat lost in conventional bulbs, the superbulbs consume much less electricity. A 100-watt superbulb draws on 40 watts, with no loss in brightness.

brightness of 100-watt bulbs. Nationally, the superbulbs would account for an energy savings of 240 billion kilowatt-hours a year, or the daily equivalent of more than half the amount of energy provided by the Alaskan pipeline.

Scientists at the Massachusetts Institute of Technology's Lincoln Laboratories have already developed the essential part of the superbulb — a transparent film or coating that is applied to the bulb's inner surface to trap heat inside the glass. In an ordinary light bulb, about 90 percent of the wattage is lost as heat (infrared radiation). The new coating conserves this heat by reflecting the infrared radiation off the bulb's inner surface and back to a centrally positioned film filament. This greatly reduces the amount of electricity needed to keep the filament hot and operating at its most efficient temperature. (The filament in a superbulb must be precisely centered in order to capture the maximum amount of reflected radiation.)

The MIT coating combines two elements in a sandwich effect: silver between two strips of titanium oxide. The coating is transparent to visible light but reflects infrared light. The scientists have perfected a method for adapting the coating to the inside of bulbs, and the Duro-Test Corporation is developing the centrally positioned filament. Superbulbs are expected to be commercially available by 1981; they will cost about twice as much as conventional light bulbs. But the savings in electricity should more than offset the difference. The energy-saving bulbs will have a life of at least 2500 hours compared with lifetimes of 750 to 1000 hours for conventional bulbs. MIT scientists assert that the energy-saving bulbs will revolutionize the lighting industry by the end of this decade.

Smart Rooms

During the 1980s scientists also plan to introduce another energy-saving device designed especially for people who forget to turn off the lights in homes and offices. Two firms are developing scanning electronic sensors that would monitor the presence of people in a room. A room installed with people sensors — called a "smart room" — would automatically turn lights on for the first person who entered the room, and turn lights off for the last person leaving the room.

22

Transportation Breakthroughs:
How You'll Get Around
Faster, Safer, and Cheaper

Future Planes

The next generation of commercial airplanes, expected to begin operations in the early 1980s, will be squatter, less fuel-thirsty, and more fully computerized. These planes will climb more effortlessly and cruise quietly, and their improved stability at lower speeds will contribute to smoother landings and greater safety. Most of these improvements will be made possible as the result of three technological breakthroughs: lightweight onboard computers, the fuel-saving high by-pass engine, and a new supercritical wing design that reduces aerodynamic drag.

Onboard Computers

Advances in microelectronics will permit the planes of the 1980s and 1990s to fly — and land — by themselves. Lightweight onboard computers will be programed with entire prearranged flight plans, as well as the best alternate plans in case of bad weather. All the calculations, including throttle settings, course headings, and descent instructions, will be decided instantly by computers instead of flight navigation engineers. While the plane is airborne, the computers will also continuously analyze each engine's performance and fuel consumption, providing the crew with constant feedback on the flight's status. The dashboard clutter of bobbing indicators and dozens of dials will be replaced by a concise digital read-out panel; one indicator will even signal bad weather ahead and the length of time left before the plane encounters it.

Improving safety is a major concern of aerodynamic engineers. They're designing the new systems to alert pilots quickly to potential dangers. For example, if a malfunction occurs, an alarm in the cockpit will alert the crew members, who will consult a special master panel referred to as the enunciator. It will provide an instant diagnosis of the problem and suggest the best remedy. Encased in this digital instrument panel will be a tiny television screen on which the pilot can study the plane's maneuvers. As the plane approaches the airport, a preprogramed diagram of that airport's runways will flash on the screen, and a dot of light will guide the pilot through his landing. The most revolutionary machine in this new safety equipment is a sophisticated instrument called the Time Reference Scanning Beam Microwave Landing System (or MLS for short), which will enable planes to land themselves in extreme low-visibility weather, or in the event that the pilot and co-pilot are incapacitated. (See *Safer Landings*, p. 279.)

High By-Pass Engine

Adopting the fuel-saving philosophy of the car industry, aviation engineers have already designed a new engine that is lighter, quieter, and burns 7 percent less fuel. This high by-pass engine sucks huge amounts of air into a central compressor and ejects it under high pressure into a combustion chamber. This dense air is sprayed with kerosene and ignited, exploding at a temperature of 2400° Farenheit. Exhaust from the explosion exits as thrust, and the force of the explosion spins a turbine that turns a huge multiblade fan at the front of the engine. Operating like an old-fashioned propeller, this fan forces back tons of air for additional thrust. A ride in a plane powered by high by-pass engines should be noticeably quieter — and perhaps cheaper, since airlines expect to save millions of dollars a year in fuel costs.

Supercritical Wing

The ideal airplane wing should slice smoothly through air, creating little turbulence and great uplift. The blunt leading edges of wings presently in use, combined with their curved upper surface, create too much drag relative to the lift they generate. They also chop the air, producing undesirable turbulence. An ingenious solution to this problem is the newly designed supercritical wing. Developed by NASA engineers, the supercritical wing resembles a glider's wing; that is, it's flatter on top, with a thinner leading edge and more tapered trailing edge. These features combine to produce less drag and stabler flying. In addition, the new wing has a slight downward slant at its trailing edge that causes air in motion to adhere to the wing's surface longer, ensuring a smoother flight. The supercritical wings are expected to appear on new planes in the late 1980s.

• • •

There will be many spectacular new planes making their débuts before the turn of the century. These will be among the first to impress the air traveler:

New Planes	Number of Seats	Seats Abreast	Number of Engines	Year to Be Introduced
Boeing 757	162–186	6	2	Spring 1982
Boeing 767	197–220	7	2	Mid 1982
Boeing 777	200–220	7	3	After 1982
McDonnel-Douglas ATMR-2	166–200	6	2	1982
Lockheed L-1011-400	220–230	9	3	1981
Airbus A310	195–245	8	2	Early 1983
British Aerospace 146	80–110	6	4	Summer 1982

Safer Landings

Air traffic is expected to double by 1985, placing an increasing burden on air traffic controllers and creating a dangerous situation for passengers, as well as for people on the ground below. Air space in the vicinity of airports is of particular concern to safety authorities, for the current Instrument Landing System (ILS) used by pilots in low-visibility weather is inadequate to handle any increase in air traffic. The dramatic solution to the safety problem resides in the Microwave Landing System (MLS), which is scheduled to replace the ILS at commercial airports over the next two decades. The system should eliminate massive traffic jams, allowing planes safely to execute complete instrument landings in zero-visibility weather.

The advantages of the MLS are best appreciated by comparing it with the ILS, the navigational system used during the last thirty years. From the ground, the ILS transmits a narrow electronic beam 6 degrees wide by 1.4 degrees high that guides planes gradually to the runway. In order to land, pilots must locate and lock onto this beam when they are about eight miles from the airport. They then must fly through the beam's narrow "funnel" single file, three minutes apart. The beam's relatively low-frequency signals are easily obstructed by tall buildings and mountains, so planes and vehicles on the ground can create false "ghost reflections," which easily confuse pilots.

By contrast, the new MLS creates a broad electronic funnel with a gaping mouth as much as 120 degrees wide by 20 degrees high. An antenna on the airplane intercepts these sweeping ground signals, and an onboard computer determines precisely where the plane is located in the funnel. Approaching aircraft can enter this funnel from many directions, at different speeds, and flying various curved paths toward separate electronic "gates"; they are guided onto the runway as close as forty seconds apart. On their computer screens, air traffic controllers and pilots will have a superior view of all the activity in the vicinity of the airport. Because MLS operates at higher radio frequences than does ILS, it is less influenced by tall structures and local geography, and its beam can cut through fog even though the fog is dense enough to prevent the pilot from seeing the nose of the plane.

MLS offers bonuses for everyone. By eliminating the need for holding patterns, thus reducing flight delays, MLS will save passengers time, and airlines fuel and money. This system will substantially reduce the concentration of noise over any neighborhood in the vicinity of an airport, because pilots will not have to fly the same path to a runway repeatedly, as they must with ILS. And for pilots forced to execute instrument landings in bad weather, MLS offers the far safer alternative of "hands-off landings," in which planes equipped with onboard computers and MLS receivers land themselves. Presently, only certain jumbo jets can perform hands-off landings, and at only the largest airports. In ten to fifteen years MLS will make it possible for all planes to be electronically landed at any airport.

The International Civil Aviation Organization approved the Time Reference Scanning Beam Microwave Landing System in 1979 for worldwide use beginning in the early 1980s. New planes coming into service this decade will be equipped with MLS instrumentation, but the cost of ground-based MLS equipment — which can run as high as $400,000 — will mean that only major

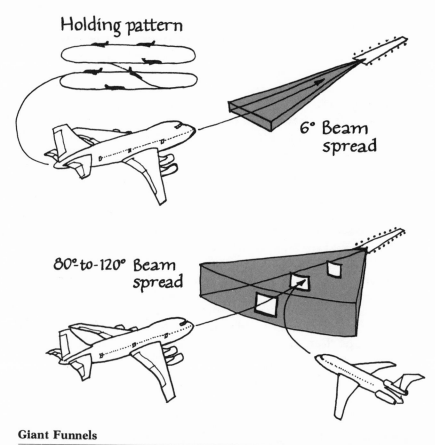

Holding pattern

6° Beam
spread

80°-to-120° Beam
spread

Giant Funnels

The increased capacity of Microwave Landing Systems to handle large numbers of planes could eliminate holding-pattern delays during peak travel hours.

airports will install the safety radar at first. They will be followed years later by smaller facilities. The Federal Aviation Authority predicts that by 1995 there should be 1600 MLS installations in the United States alone. MLS is a technology breakthrough that promises to keep the friendly skies friendly and maintain air travel as the safest way to travel.

Electric Cars

An all electric-powered car that can be driven at speeds up to 60 miles an hour, travel 300 miles without recharging, and recharge in little more time than it takes to fill a car's gas tank — all for about the same cost as a gas-powered car — is only about two decades away. The production of such electric cars awaits the perfection of the superbattery, which, unlike its predecessor, the lead-acid battery, will be lightweight in relation to the amount of power it delivers.

The technology required to develop superbatteries is extremely complex. For superbatteries to be practical and economical, they must produce considerable amounts of electric power and have a cycle lifetime (the number of times or cycles a battery can be recharged) of at least two to three years. In additon, superbatteries must be safe. To attain the first two of these criteria, the chemical ingredients in a superbattery should, in theory, operate at temperatures of several hundred degrees, react violently with each other, and be highly corrosive to everything but their containers. Yet because of these optimum properties, superbatteries are potential killers for motorists who may be involved in accidents with electric cars.

Nevertheless, researchers are making impressive headway developing superbatteries and minimizing their dangers. The United States Department of Energy recently awarded $26 million to several companies and universities to continue work on perfecting a variety of superbatteries that show particular promise.

Sodium-Sulfur Battery

Simply put, a battery is an electrochemical device for converting chemical energy into electrical energy. The active electrochemical materials, known as a couple, form the negative (anode) and positive (cathode) terminals, and interact through a medium called an electrolyte. (In the conventional lead-acid battery, lead and lead dioxide form the couple, and the electrolyte is sulfuric acid.) The major requirement of a couple is that one member must be able easily to release electrically charged particles (electrons or ions), and the other member must be able to collect these particles, producing an electric current.

One promising couple being developed by the Dow Chemical Company in the United States and the Chloride Company in England combines liquid sodium (the anode) and liquid sulfur (the cathode), separated by a solid partition (the electrolyte). A sodium-sulfur battery, which must operate in the temperature range of 570° to 660° Fahrenheit, theoretically can deliver 6.3 times more power per pound of battery than the conventional lead-acid battery. In the 1960s, the Ford Motor Company tested an early model of a sodium-sulfur battery in an experimental electric car. The car ran slowly, had poor acceleration, and didn't travel very far before the battery died. Ford scientists also learned that if the partition separating the two hot liquids cracked, the battery would, in effect, be transformed into a bomb.

Scientists at the Chloride Company report better luck. They've designed a sodium-sulfur battery that uses a durable ceramic cylinder for the partition between the potentially explosive liquids. Sodium is contained inside the ceramic; sulfur remains on the outside. The battery maintains its required operating temperature with self-contained heating coils. (In Dow Chemical's successful new design, the all-critical partition is ultrathin, insulated boron glass.) This exotic superbattery is expected to cost about the same per unit of energy it delivers as a good lead-acid battery, and it should have a life of well over 3000 charge-discharge cycles.

Sodium-sulfur batteries will be tested in cars, trucks, and industrial equipment in the early 1980s. Although scientists are taking great precautions to insulate the batteries in case of accidents, the fact remains that molten sodium and sulfur are explosive on contact. In the long run, that knowledge is expected to affect the public's reaction to this particular breed of superbattery. Many scientists feel that sodium-sulfur batteries must prove their safety through a decade of use in industrial applications before the public will accept them in electric-powered cars.

Lithium–Metal Sulfide Battery

At least four American companies are working on versions of this battery. Theoretically, it has the potential to store 7.2 times more power per pound of battery than lead-acid batteries. In the most common version of this superbattery, lithium (alloyed with aluminum) serves as the anode, and an iron sulfide cathode operates in an electrolytic mixture of lithium chloride and potassium chloride. To generate its maximum output of electric current, however, a lithium–iron sulfide battery must operate in the extreme temperature range of 700° to 840° Fahrenheit.

Currently lithium–iron sulfide batteries are prohibitively expensive, and their performance is only beginning to be tested in laboratories. Nevertheless, their potential to produce electric energy is alluring. Eagle Picher Industries is building a lithium battery that will be tested in vehicles by scientists at Argonne National Laboratories in 1981. General Motors scientists are researching their own complex version of a lithium battery that has produced electric power for 5000 hours in laboratory tests.

GM scientists predict their lithium batteries eventually will be able to power electric cars for 200 miles before they need recharging.

Despite high internal-operating temperatures, a commercial lithium battery would not be hot to touch. And unlike the sodium-sulfur battery, a crack in a lithium–iron sulfide battery would produce not an explosion but a stream of molten chemicals that should prove fairly easy to contain. Lithium batteries possess such a tremendous power potential that scientists are determined to perfect them, lower their cost, and design them safely.

Zinc-Chloride Battery

This is an exotic superbattery that has already been successfully tested in various electric cars and trucks. Most recently, a zinc-chloride battery developed by Energy Development Associates of Michigan powered a Chevrolet Vega at normal highway speeds for 200 miles on a single charge.

A zinc-chloride battery is slightly less powerful than either the sodium-sulfur or lithium–iron sulfide battery, but it possesses three highly desirable qualities: it runs at normal ambient temperatures; its electrolyte is an inexpensive solution of zinc chloride and water; and it does not produce a chemical action while a car is idle. The zinc-chloride battery's most serious drawback is that its chief ingredient, chlorine, is a deadly gas at ambient temperatures. In attempts to overcome this potential danger, scientists have devised a method for storing the chlorine in a solid state (as chlorine hydrate) while the battery is idle. During operation, heat from the battery converts measured amounts of solid chlorine to gas as it's needed to produce electricity. This greatly minimizes the amount of chlorine gas that would escape if a crack developed in the battery. Still, if a car powered by a zinc-chloride battery was involved in a collision, heat resulting from friction or fire could, presumably, vaporize the deadly chlorine. Research is continuing on zinc-chloride batteries, but, once again, it will be the public who ultimately decides to risk driving electric cars powered by batteries that may be dangerous.

Fuel Cells

These devices are similar in structure to batteries but vary in fundamental operation. Fuel cells have been used widely in spacecraft, and they have the potential for generating several hundred

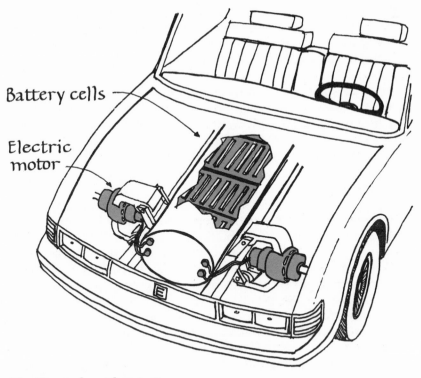

Battery cells

Electric motor

The Heart of an Electric Car

A major challenge facing engineers is to design superbatteries that produce abundant electric power yet are safe in case of automobile collisions.

times the electric power of even the best superbatteries currently being developed.

A fuel cell consists of positive and negative electrodes separated by an electrolyte that transmits ions but not electrons. As its name implies, a fuel cell "burns" fuel. That is, it combines the fuel it is using with oxygen to produce electricity — and this process is free of the usual pollutants. There are as many different kinds of fuel cells as there are fuels that react vigorously with oxygen. Fuel cells in a spacecraft, for instance, combine hydrogen with oxygen to produce electricity. Most fuel cells operate at relatively low temperatures of 70° to 120° Celsius. A fuel cell's greatest appeal lies in the fact that as long as it is fed an ample supply of its particular kind of fuel — and water — it will continue to produce clean electricity without having to be recharged.

Scientists at Lockheed are developing a lithium fuel cell that in fifteen years may be able to power a standard-size car for 300 miles. Such a car would have to stop for servicing about every 200 to 300 miles to have fresh water added to its battery and to have the battery's reaction by-product — dry, powderlike lithium carbonate — removed. New metal-lithium plates inserted into slots in the fuel cell system would restore the battery's initial power. The lithium-carbonate by-product would be collected by service stations and recycled for metal-lithium plates.

Fuel cell technology already exists. In addition to using fuel cells in spacecraft, several utility companies are constructing full-scale fuel cell power plants consisting of huge stacks of several hundred fuel cells; these could provide substantial amounts of electricity for urban and metropolitan areas. A 4.5-megawatt plant, for instance, will be built in New York City in the early 1980s. However, the use of fuel cells to power electric cars presents a major challenge to researchers; the fuel cell system has to be powerful, yet sufficiently small and lightweight to fit under the hood of a car. Scientists predict it will take ten years to produce such a compact high–energy density system, and perhaps another ten years to test the system and incorporate it into automobile design. Electric cars powered by fuel cells are not expected to be on the road until the early part of the next century.

Car Sonar

One method for improving the safety of superbattery-powered electric cars is equipping them with sonar systems that would prevent rear-end collisions, the most common of automobile accidents. Two American companies are already working on the design for sonar auto units. According to the companies, one unit would be concealed in the front grill of a car, and the second unit would be installed in the trunk. While the car is running, the sonar devices would continually emit signals, which, in turn, would bounce off vehicles both immediately behind and ahead of the sonar-equipped car. A minicomputer in the car would work on the Doppler principle to measure the change in reflected sound frequencies, continually calculating the distance of the nearest cars and registering that distance in feet on a digital panel.

A motorist could set the sonar device alarm to guide him in maintaining safe distances. Any car approaching within this preset sonar boundary would trigger a flashing light on the dashboard or sound a buzzer. This alarm would be of great aid in preventing accidents, especially when you consider the United States Department of Highway Safety statistic that most rear-end collisions occur because drivers are either preoccupied with conversation or daydreaming and don't realize how closely they are tailgating until it's too late. A buzzer would alert these drivers in time to avoid accidents. In addition, car sonar could come in handy for determining clearances when you're trying to park in tight spaces. Automobile sonar units should be commercially available by the mid 1980s.

Levitating Trains

Trains are expected to make a major comeback with the advent of magnetically levitated trains, or Maglevs. These new trains may even rival airplanes as the dominant form of intermediate-distance travel in the future. Offering smooth, silent rides over even the roughest terrain, the Maglevs will float above a U-curved aluminum track, levitated by supercooled magnets. The first Maglev trains — which could be in operation in the United States by the mid 1990s (and in Japan as early as 1983) — could travel above ground at several hundred miles an hour, but eventually they may whisk through vacuum tunnels at speeds up to 1300 miles an hour.

A few years ago an experimental 600-pound Maglev train, measuring 3 feet by 14 feet, was tested by engineers at California's Stanford Research Institute. Although it was a primitive prototype that lifted only a few inches off its track and traveled a mere 250 feet, its performance convinced scientists that the principle behind Maglev trains is practical. That principle, of course, is that like magnetic polarities repel, and dissimilar magnetic polarities attract.

With research funded by the United States Department of Energy, the Ford Motor Company, the Massachusetts Institute of Technology, and the Rand Corporation are all developing various magnetic levitation systems.

The future Maglev train will be designed with powerful electromagnets mounted on its bullet-shaped body. The electromagnets will be cooled to $-450°$ Fahrenheit by liquid helium stored in tanks under the train's floor. When an electric current is passed through the magnets, the train will lift about ten inches off its track and be pulled forward by an attraction to the opposite magnetic polarity lying in the track ahead of it. Since supercooled electromagnets offer virtually no resistance to electric current,

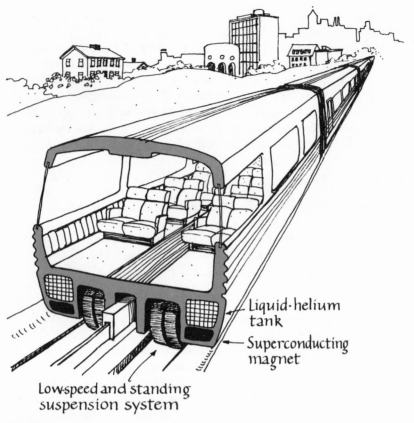

Liquid-helium tank

Superconducting magnet

Low-speed and standing suspension system

Rapid Transit

No longer a dream, experimental magnetically levitated trains are being tested, and the first commercial Maglevs may be operating in Japan by 1983.

the initial current used to float a train will continue to circulate undiminished, buoying the train with no need for additional power, though a small amount of energy is constantly required to keep the liquid helium supercooled.

Theoretically, Maglev trains have a significant advantage over airplanes. The aerodynamic drag due to friction between a plane and ambient air increases with the airplane's speed, but the magnetic drag between a Maglev train and its track peaks quickly as the train accelerates from rest, and then actually decreases with speed.

Because the Maglev trains of the 1990s will travel aboveground, their speed will be limited to about 300 miles an hour, but the Maglev trains of the first quarter of the next century will travel much faster through vacuum tunnels that offer little or no air resistance. The Rand Corporation has already researched the feasibility of building partly air-tight tunnels and estimates that construction costs may run $50 million for every mile of tunnel. That enormous cost is expected to be offset by the flood of revenue generated by the speedy and inexpensive-to-operate trains. An underground Maglev train could complete a New York–Los Angeles run in less than a half-hour — and for a fare as reasonable as $50. That's the kind of service that may eventually encourage us to abandon our cars in favor of mass transit. At least, this is what the United States Department of Energy officials are hoping for. They have elevated research of the Maglev trains to one of their top priority goals for the future.

Endless Trains

Though you may ride on a Maglev train cross-country, there's a good chance that early in the next century you may shuttle quickly around your own city on "endless" trains that are arranged in continuous loops.

Endless trains are the brainchild of Lawrence Bell, professor of industrial design at the University of Illinois. They are closed loop conveyors — Bell has titled them Synchroveyor Urban Mass Transportation Systems — that can transport passengers at speeds up to thirty miles an hour.

A synchroveyer, for instance, could circle a city's downtown area. Passengers would board or disembark the conveyor at intervals of forty to ninety seconds. They could also transfer between adjacent loops: when two endless trains were traveling at the same speed, passengers would step onto a transfer deck between the adjacent loops and the deck would revolve, letting them step from one loop (or train) to the other.

Though Professor Bell's endless train is still on the drawing board, the technical know-how to build such a system exists. With the increased necessity for mass transit in metropolitan areas, endless trains may be transporting large numbers of people in heavily populated areas by the early part of the next century. If so, cars may become a rarity on city streets, and city dwellers may have the luxury of living in less congested, unpolluted, more pleasant urban environments.

23

Space Breakthroughs:
Colonizing Space–and the Search for Extraterrestrial Life

Space Homes

An earthlike space colony landscaped with parks, lakes, and mountains to house thousands of people could be orbiting our world by the year 2000. The inhabitants would enjoy a pollution- and pest-free environment and control their own weather. They may even ride the space shuttle once a year to vacation on earth. These first space colonists could quickly repay the enormous $90 million cost of their interplanetary city by mining ores on the moon; manufacturing perfect machine parts, pure alloys, and drugs in the near-zero-gravity vacuum of space; and by erecting solar power satellites that would beam inexpensive, plentiful solar energy back to earth in the form of microwaves. By the year 2150, some scientists believe, more people could be living in orbiting space colonies than on earth.

At any rate, this is the visionary goal of Princeton University physicist Dr. Gerard O'Neill. Many top scientists support O'Neill's plan, and exobiologist Carl Sagan, testifying before a government committee considering the feasibility of space colonization, has said, "Our technology is capable of extraordinary new ventures in space, one of which is the space city idea . . . That's an extremely expensive undertaking, but it seems to be historically of the greatest significance."

O'Neill has calculated that the most favorable location in space to construct colonies is a region of stable gravity equidistant from both the earth and moon. Each colony, or island, would slowly rotate to simulate the effects of earth's gravity. According to O'Neill, Island One would be of modest size, having a diameter of 1500 feet, weighing three million tons, and would serve as home for 10,000 people. Four thousand people would be engaged in building Island Two, while 6000 mined the moon and constructed solar power satellites for earth's energy needs.

A space colony would not only be homey; it would be a healthy, enjoyable place to live, claims O'Neill.

The interior of the colony would be as earth-like as possible — rich in green plants, trees, animals, birds . . . The design would allow a line of sight of at least a half mile, giving the residents a feeling of spaciousness. Residential areas might consist of small apartment buildings with big rooms and wide terraces overlooking fields and groves. Near the axis of the structure, gravity would be much reduced and, consequently, human-powered flight would be easy, sports and ballet could take on a new dimension and weight would almost disappear. It seems almost a certainty that at such a level a person with a serious heart condition could live far longer than on earth, and that low gravity could greatly ease many of the health problems of advancing age.

Space Agriculture

Future colonies would be bigger. Island Three, for example, would be four miles across, possess twenty-mile-long extensions (suburbs), house a population of several million people, and contain a controlled environment superior to earth's. The colony would have separate residential, agricultural, and industrial areas, each with its ideal gravity and climate. Many of the colonists would be trained as contemporary farmers. By opening and closing huge aluminum shades facing the sun, these farmers could tailor the length of a day and growing season to suit particular crops. And in the pest-free environment space agriculture would be profitable and its annual yields predictable. For Island One, claims O'Neill, "only 111 acres would be needed to feed all 10,000 residents."

Unlike earth's delicate biosphere, which is continually threatened by manmade heat and energy, the cold void of space would absorb all the waste heat generated by the colony. Supporting O'Neill's scheme, science writer Isaac Asimov told the House Subcommittee on Space Science and Applications, "It is my opinion that the important goal for space exploration over the next century is the establishment of an ecologically independent human colony on the Moon, or on artificial space colonies that use the Moon as a quarry for raw material." O'Neill adds: "The human race stands now on the threshold of a new frontier whose richness is a thousand times greater than that of the new western world of 500 years ago."

Will space colonies actually be constructed?

Most scientists agree that the colonization of space is inevitable and that O'Neill's designs for space homes are realistic. But they claim that O'Neill's timetable for the exodus into space is far too optimistic and that we can't begin to construct a timetable until the space shuttle commences regular flights and engineers determine how easy (or difficult) it is to transport materials into space and to perform construction in zero-gravity.

Scientists expect to have much of this kind of information by the end of the 1980s. In the meantime, NASA has appropriated funds to investigate further the feasibility of space colonization. What we have to gain technically and socially from a concerted effort to colonize space was convincingly described by Isaac Asimov to the House Subcommittee:

• Observatories beyond Earth's atmosphere can lead to a better knowledge of the Universe and the laws of nature governing it — with unpredictable but surely great applications to the human way of life.

• The presence of infinite amounts of hard vacuum, of low temperatures, of high solar radiation, should make possible industrial activities of types not practical on Earth, leading to unpredictable but surely great advances in technology.

• The establishment of a working colony, ecologically independent, on either the Moon or in an artificial structure in space will require a society fundamentally different from our own — a society that can live in an engineered environment under conditions of strict recycling and mineral waste. Since this is precisely the sort of condition toward which terrestrial life is tending, the colonies will serve as schools to Earth, as experiments in living from which we may profit immensely.

• The establishment of a colony will be difficult enough and expensive enough to require a global — rather than a national — effort. The effort will be great enough to supply mankind with a common goal and a common sense of pride that may transcend local chauvinisms, and thus encourage the growth of a global political community — and indeed serve as a substitute for the emotional catharsis of war.

• Lunar or space colonists, living in engineered worlds, on the inside, would be more psychologically adapted to life in a spaceship undertak-

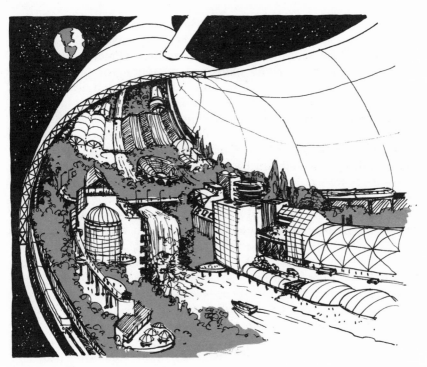

Life in Orbit

Landscaped, for nostalgic reasons, to resemble the earth, this space habitat for 10,000 people would rotate about its axis to simulate earth's gravity. By opening and closing huge aluminum panels, the colony's farmers could tailor the length of days or seasons to optimize agricultural yields.

ing long voyages, so it will be by them rather than Earthmen that the rest of the Solar System (and eventually the stars perhaps) will be explored.

• Colonies in space generally will supply a chance for growth and adventure after Earth itself has, perforce, adopted a no-growth philosophy.

Our First Close Encounter

NASA has outlined an enormous plan to search with radio telescopes for evidence of extraterrestrial intelligence (ETI) during the 1980s and 1990s. Cornell University astronomer Frank Drake gives the program a fifty-fifty chance of success, and Carl Sagan asserts that contact with aliens may be achieved within our lifetime.

Few astronomers are quite as optimistic as Drake and Sagan, but most consider communications with ETI (CETI) a genuine possibility. They claim there may be a million planets suitable for life within our Milky Way galaxy alone. They point to the fact that in the last two decades radio astronomers have detected more than forty organic molecules in interstellar space, including carbon monoxide, formaldehyde, and hydrogen cyanide, one probable triumvirate that may have been the precursor of the chemical components of terrestrial life. Drake thinks "there is almost nothing you can do to stop a primitive atmosphere from making the molecules of life." Exobiologists agree that the search for ETI (SETI) — pointing our electronic ears in precisely the right direction at the right time — involves sheer luck, but the rewards will be extraordinary. Contact with aliens would profoundly affect our life materially, as well as philosophically and spiritually. An advanced civilization, for instance, may teach us how to extend life, eliminate disease, and avoid nuclear and environmental disaster.

The attempts to search for ETI began in 1960 when Frank Drake used radio telescopes at the National Radio Astronomy Observatory in Green Bank, Virginia. Since then there have been over a dozen searches by Soviet, British, Canadian, and American astronomers. Since 1975 the powerful electronic ear at Arecibo in Puerto Rico has eavesdropped on five close galaxies, earth's nearest 200 stars, and even beamed out its own Hello! — a burst of energy ten million times brighter than the sun — which caused Drake, who sent the message, to comment, "For three minutes we became the brightest star in our galaxy."

Pioneers 10 and 11 have already carried plaques etched with human images and details of our science and solar system past Jupiter; they will skirt Saturn in 1980 and then leave the solar system for eons of galactic travel. Voyagers 1 and 2 each carry a gold-plated copper record in an aluminum jacket containing samples of earth languages from English to Esperanto: music from Bach to bagpipes ("Earth's greatest hits," as Drake refers to them); sounds of earthquakes, thunder, wind, and rain; calls of hyenas, whales, and human infants; the beat of a human heart and a hearty burst of human laughter; plus coded pictures in color and black and white of DNA, the human anatomy, plants, flowers, conception, birth, and most of your other favorite topics. Sagan, the imaginative force behind these endeavors, admits that the likelihood of such a message being intercepted is almost zero, but without the effort, he argues, the chance for contact is absolutely zero. (Unless, of course, *they* take the initiative to contact *us*.) With the 1980s comes the most ambitious endeavor of all — Project SETI — which Drake and Sagan hope will lead to CETI. (ETI, SETI, and CETI are acronyms we may as well get accustomed to because they are going to fill the pages of newspapers and magazines over the next few decades.)

Listening for Aliens in the 1980s and 1990s

If funding for Project SETI is soon appropriated, the search for ETI could start by the mid 1980s. Three big radio telescopes, including the one at Arecibo, focus on sunlike stars a few hundred light-years from earth, perhaps listening to each one for thirty minutes each night. At the same time the Goldstone radio telescope in the Mojave Desert would listen over a broader range of frequencies for ETI voices of higher and lower register. Next, Project SETI calls for construction of a huge radio receiver that can tune into one million channels and increase the odds of picking up signals. And by 1990 NASA may have built its ultimate dream ear: a multimillion-dollar Cyclops, a mammoth array of 1500 radio dishes, each 100 meters across, gathered in a tight circle. From space, Cyclops will resemble a field of shiny silver and white daisies.

Project SETI is the brain child of astronomers at NASA's Ames Research Center in Mountain View, California, and the Jet Propulsion Laboratory in Pasadena. Ames astronomers would man the Arecibo antenna, and the Goldstone dish would be operated by the JPL team. They are already envisioning an alternative to the costly ground-based Cyclops: a huge orbiting receiving dish that would be launched into space by the shuttle, to collect signals and relay them to earth. Project scientists have compelling reasons to believe that life in space will also be based on carbon compounds (the next most likely life–building blocks are silicon and boron). Since the most efficient way to survey the electromagnetic environment that permeates the universe is with "eyes," exobiologists feel that ETIs will probably have eyes — perhaps ones sensitive to the radio, infrared, ultraviolet, and X-ray portions of the spectrum, as well as to the visible portions.

But eavesdropping can work two ways. Some thirty years of our television and radio signals, plus the infrared heat radiated by industry and daily living, should make it easy for an advanced civilization to detect our presence. Drake has calculated that the waves from our TV and radio programs, traveling at the speed of

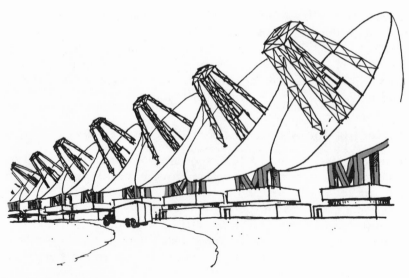

Earth's Largest Ear

Cyclops, the proposed array of fifteen hundred 100-meter dish antennas, would listen for evidence of extraterrestrial intelligence in the 1990s. Conversely, thirty years of our television and radio programs, traveling through space, may currently be falling on similar electronic ears on other planets — challenging extraterrestrial sociologists to decipher the seemingly bizarre nature of life on earth.

light, have now sped past some 400 suns, their planets, and their inhabitants, if they exist. He claims that intelligent signals from other civilizations are impinging on us right now, but they're simply too weak for our present equipment to detect, or perhaps we don't know which channel to tune to. This particular problem is what Project SETI could remedy, if the program is ultimately approved by Congress.

The hope of the project scientists during the next two decades is clearly stated in SETI's report:

Were we to locate but a single extraterrestrial signal, we would know immediately one great truth: that it is possible for a civilization to maintain an advanced technological state and not destroy itself. We might even learn that life and intelligence pervade the Universe . . . [We might learn] all sorts of scientific results, ranging from a valid picture of the past and the future of the Universe through theories of the fundamental particles to whole new biologies. Some conjecture that we might hear from near-immortals the views of distant and venerable thinkers on the deepest values of conscious beings and their societies! Perhaps we will forever become linked with a chain of rich cultures, a vast galactic network. Who can say?

What we can say is this: moviegoers have shelled out $100 million to see a fantasy close encounter of the third kind. For the same price we may experience a close encounter of the real kind — and in our lifetime.

Notes

Notes

1. HOLISTIC HEALTH BREAKTHROUGHS

4 "The studies indicate . . ." Jerome D. Frank, "The Medical Power of Faith," *Human Nature*, August 1978, p. 45. Dr. Frank's article presents an excellent overview of the role of drugs and environment in mind-body healing, as does his slightly more technical paper, "Mind-Body Relationship In Illness and Healing," *Journal of the International Academy of Preventive Medicine*, vol. 2, no. 3, 1977. The examples I have cited of mind-body interactions are from these sources.

5 "State of mind may well account . . ." "The Medical Power of Faith," *Human Nature*, p. 44.

5 "We have seen the importance . . ." Ibid., p. 47.

9 The cancer case related by Dr. Bruno Klopfer is recounted in Constance Holden, "Cancer and the Mind: How Are They Connected?" *Science*, vol. 200, June 1978, p. 1369.

11 "First we must understand . . ." "Heart attacks from stress via brain," *Science News*, vol. 114, no. 21, November 18, 1978, p. 342.

2. NUTRITION BREAKTHROUGHS

12 "Every individual has . . ." Roger J. Williams, "Nutritional Individuality," *Human Nature*, June 1978, p. 46. Nutritional statistics cited in this section are from this source, as well as from a comprehensive article by Sam Keen, et al., "Food and Consciousness," *Psychology Today*, pp. 62–94. Dr. Williams' dietary recommendations can be found in this reference.

15 "Higher levels of these chemicals . . ." Richard Wurtman, "The Brain," *Psychology Today*, October 1978, p. 140.

15 "It is a complete surprise . . ." Ibid.
16 "Although tryptophan . . ." Ernest Hartmann, "L-Tryptophan — The Sleeping Pill of the Future?" *Psychology Today*, December 1978, p. 180.
16 "is to eat a high-carbohydrate . . ." Wurtman, op. cit.
18 "Combined with the animal studies . . ." Connie Bruck, "Vitamins," *New Times*, July 24, 1978, p. 59.
19 "Evolution took place . . ." "Vitamins," Ibid., p. 62.
20 "B-15 seems to have . . ." Lee Torrey, "When is a vitamin a non-fuel nutrient?" *New Scientist*, June 1, 1978, p. 573.

3. CANCER BREAKTHROUGHS
27 "It is clear that selenium . . ." From a report to the National Cancer Institute by Pietro Gullino, 1978.
35 "We think that our studies . . ." Harold M. Schmeck, Jr., "Interferon Curbs Cancer in Three Cases," *New York Times*, January 6, 1979.

4. HEART BREAKTHROUGHS
41 "The really important question . . ." Jane E. Brody, "Study Links Eggs to Increase in Cholesterol-carrying Protein," *New York Times*, November 8, 1978.
45 "abstinence from alcohol . . ." William J. Darby, "The Benefits of Drink," *Human Nature*, November 1978, pp. 31–37.
45 Dr. Darby's definitions of a drink, as well as the statistics in this section, are in his excellent survey article cited above.
48 "This gives the person . . ." Obtained in a personal interview with Dr. Kenneth Greenspan.

6. TREATMENT BREAKTHROUGHS
62 The statistics on the amounts of trace elements in hair are cited by Thomas H. Maugh II, "Hair: A Diagnostic Tool to Complement Blood Serum and Urine," *Science*, vol. 202, December 22, 1978, pp. 1271–1273.
69 *Awakening the Dead.* Information and quotations in this section are from an interview with Dr. Arnold Starr and from *Newsweek*, June 10, 1974, p. 56. "In several cases where the patient appears to be . . ." is from George Getze, "A New Way to Detect Brain Death," New York *Post*, November 17, 1975.

7. GENE BREAKTHROUGHS
71 "The isolation of genes . . ." Ted Howard and Jeremy Rifkin, *Who Should Play God?* (New York: Dell, 1977), p. 28.
75 "avoid occupations such as . . ." Tabitha Powledge, "Can genetic screening prevent occupational disease?" *New Scientist*, September 2, 1976, p. 487.
75 "It is now conceivable that . . ." Howard and Rifkin, op. cit., p. 147.
77 "might appreciably affect the overall quality . . ." Ibid., p. 148.
79 "The ultimate impact . . ." *Business Week*, August 9, 1976, p. 67.

80 "This is a long-range technology . . ." Dan Hager, "The New Botany," *TWA Ambassador*, May 1978, p. 48.

80 "The fusion process was fairly simple . . ." Press release, "Tobacco Plant Fused with Human Tumor Cells," Brookhaven National Laboratory, July 29, 1976.

8. INFERTILITY BREAKTHROUGHS

92 "It is conceivable that an embryo . . ." Julie Ann Miller, "Cells On Ice," *Science News*, vol. 114, no. 12, September 16, 1978, p. 206.

9. FEMALE HEALTH BREAKTHROUGHS

96 "The women's liberation movement . . ." Obtained in a personal interview with Dr. Kenneth Greenspan.

101 "There is little doubt that . . ." *The Lancet*, June 10, 1978, p. 1223.

10. BIORHYTHM BREAKTHROUGHS

109 "This shows that mental ability . . ." "Jensen: Intelligence a 'Biological Rhythm,'" *Science News*, vol. 114, no. 11, September 9, 1978, p. 181.

110 "These people suffer . . ." Obtained in an interview with Dr. Charles Pollak.

111 "maybe people (with affective disorders) . . ." Joel Greenberg, "Cracking the Cycles of Depression and Mania," *Science News*, vol. 114, no. 22, November 25, 1978, p. 367.

112 "We have to be very careful . . ." Ibid., p. 367.

11. BRAIN BREAKTHROUGHS

117 "One's environment, particularly early life . . ." "Human Aggression Linked to Chemical Balance," *Science News*, vol. 113, no. 22, June 3, 1978, p. 356.

119 "There is very little doubt . . ." "Endorphins for emotions: A good beta," *Science News*, vol. 114, no. 20, November 11, 1978, p. 326.

121 "have either gotten well or improved . . ." "Is Schizophrenia in the Blood?" *Science News*, vol. 114, no. 2, July 8, 1978, p. 29.

127 "It will take decades . . ." Gene Bylinsky, "A Preview of the 'Choose Your Mood Society,'" *Fortune*, March 1977, p. 221. This article provides an excellent survey of the pioneering drug design research of Arnold Mandell and Alexander Shulgin.

12. SLEEP BREAKTHROUGHS

129 "This can have profound effects . . ." Obtained in an interview with Dr. Charles Pollak.

129 "There is a great desire . . ." Joel Greenberg, "The Aging of Sleep," *Science News*, vol. 114, no. 1, July 1, 1978, p. 11.

133 "You introduce a lot of facts . . ." Obtained in an interview with Dr. Chester Pearlman.

13. AGING BREAKTHROUGHS

137 "With catatoxic substances . . ." Hans Selye, "They All Looked Sick to Me," *Human Nature*, February 1978, p. 62.

139 "merely Parkinson's disease gone from . . ." "Aging: Catecholamines Lost," *Science News*, vol. 114, no. 24, December 9, 1978, p. 408.

141 "general reduction of suspicion . . ." "Cleaning the brain's tubes holds back senility," *New Scientist*, February 17, 1977, p. 395.

142 The social, political, and religious impact of anti-aging pills. Reprinted with permission from Jib Fowles, "The Transition to a Society of Immortals," *The Futurist*, June 1978 (published by the World Future Society), pp. 180–181.

14. BEHAVIOR BREAKTHROUGHS

146 *Rearing Your Baby*. Examples in this section of the awareness of newborns are cited in Adian MacFarlane, "What a Baby Knows," *Human Nature*, February 1978, pp. 74–81, and from a personal interview with Dr. Lewis Lipsitt.

148 "psychiatric concepts and techniques don't work . . ." Eugene H. Methvin, "The Criminal Mind: A Startling New Look," *Reader's Digest*, May 1978, p. 121. The complete study by Samuel Yochelson and Stanton Samenow is contained in three volumes: *The Criminal Personality*, vol. I and vol. II (Jason Aronson, publisher); vol. III should be released in the early 1980s.

15. BIOMETEOROLOGY BREAKTHROUGHS

159 "The precise date and hour . . ." *Climate and Health*, published by the National Oceanic and Atmospheric Administration, Boulder, Colorado, vol. 6, no. 4, October 1976.

161 The examples in this section, Ions for Your Health, are from Albert Krueger and Sheelah Sigel, "Ions in the Air," *Human Nature*, July 1978, pp. 46–52, and from a personal interview with Dr. Albert Krueger.

164 "We are being very cautious . . ." Krueger and Sigel, op. cit., p. 52.

16. EARTH BREAKTHROUGHS

171 "the first scientific evidence . . ." and "the animals were more restless . . ." are from a report by the Stanford Outdoor Primate Facility, 1976.

172 "Deer formed flocks . . ." "Animals' Actions Before Quakes May Be Linked to Particles in Air," *New York Times*, December 31, 1978.

172 "Documentation in China is very good . . ." "Animals Sense Change Before Quake Strikes," *Science Digest*, March 1978, p. 18.

17. WEATHER BREAKTHROUGHS

181 "One could launch boats . . ." Contained in a technical report submitted in early 1979 to the American Association for the Advancement of Science's journal, *Science*.

184 "changes in the earth's orbital geometry . . ." Richard A. Kerr, "Climate Control: How Large a Role for Orbital Variations?" *Science*, vol. 201, July 14, 1978, p. 146. In this article Kerr presents an excellent survey of recent research linking climate and variations in the earth's orbit; pages 144–146.

18. MIND-BOGGLING BREAKTHROUGHS

194 "The gravitational constant will continue . . ." Dietrick E. Thomsen, "Cosmology Against the Grain," *Science News*, vol. 114, no. 9, August 26, 1978, p. 140. This entire issue is devoted to recent discoveries in astronomy and cosmology and provides an excellent overview, in lucid, lay language, of one of the most exciting disciplines in modern science.

211 "Chances are overwhelming that the earth . . ." Quoted by Martin Gardner in *The New York Review*, November 23, 1978, p. 15.

211 "chances of the existence of man . . ." Ibid., p. 16.

19. MEDICAL TECHNOLOGY BREAKTHROUGHS

227 "With NMR the body's . . ." Susan Renner-Smith, "Damadian's Supermagnet," *Popular Science*, December 1977, p. 76.

227 "We might be able to beam . . ." Ibid., p. 78.

20. COMMUNICATIONS BREAKTHROUGHS

241 "Tomorrow's telephone will become the key . . ." Interview with Charles L. Brown in *U.S. News & World Report*, February 12, 1979, p. 63.

250 "People will be giving their opinions . . ." "TV Set Views Viewer," *New York Times*, August 8, 1978.

251 "Applications of neutrino communications . . ." Malcolm W. Browne, "A Message Through the Earth, Not Around It, Hinted Soon," *New York Times*, October 28, 1977, and Malcolm W. Browne, "Scientists Forecasting Beam Through Earth to Transmit Messages," *New York Times*, December 24, 1978.

21. ENERGY BREAKTHROUGHS

257 "We need capital investment . . ." *New York Times*, February 25, 1979.

259 "Average Wind Speed" statistics compiled by the National Weather Service and quoted in D. S. Halacy, Jr., *Earth, Water, Wind and Sun* (New York: Harper & Row, 1977), p. 106.

271 According to a prediction by the Department of Energy . . . at a cost of $120 billion! Janet Raloff, "Thermionics," *Science News*, vol. 113, no. 13, April 1, 1978, p. 202.

22. TRANSPORTATION BREAKTHROUGHS

277 *Future Planes.* The fundamental operations of onboard computers, the high by-pass engine, and supercritical wings are as described in "The 1980s Generation," *Time*, August 14, 1978, pp. 57–59.

23. SPACE BREAKTHROUGHS

290 "our technology is capable of extraordinary . . ." Quoted in Gerard
   K. O'Neill, "Space Colonies: The High Frontier," in *1999, The World
   of Tomorrow* (Washington, D.C.: World Futurist Society, 1978), p. 72.
   The book is a selection of articles from *The Futurist;* O'Neill's article
   is based on his testimony before Congress on July 23, 1975.

291 "The interior of the colony would be earth-like . . ." Ibid., p. 69.

291 "only 111 acres would be needed . . ." Ibid., p. 69.

291 "It is my opinion that the important goal . . ." Ibid., p. 69.

292 Isaac Asimov's comments to the House Subcommittee on Space
   Science and Applications are also quoted in "Space Colonies: The
   High Frontier," Ibid., p. 69.

294 "there is almost nothing you can do to stop . . ." Alton Blakesless,
   "Listening For Life," *Omni*, October 1978, p. 64.

294 "For three minutes . . ." Ibid., p. 144.

297 "Were we to locate but a single extraterrestrial signal . . ." from the
   1977 SETI report as quoted in "Listening for Life," Ibid., p. 146.